Fundamental Aspects of Gastrointestinal Nursing

Fundamental Aspects of Gastrointestinal Nursing

edited by

Carol L. Cox, Martin J. Steggall
and Alison M. Coutts

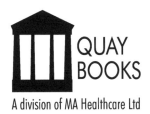

QUAY
BOOKS

A division of MA Healthcare Ltd

Quay Books Division, MA Healthcare Ltd, St Jude's Church, Dulwich Road, London
SE24 0PB

British Library Cataloguing-in-Publication Data
A catalogue record is available for this book

ISBN-10: 1 85642 426 X
ISBN-13: 978 1 85642 426 4

Printed by Mimeo, Huntingdon, Cambridgeshire

Contents

Contents

This book is dedicated to Karen Elizabeth Knowlton, loving daughter and nurse who died on 20 April 2010 of acute pancreatitis, intra-abdominal abscesses and sepsis.

Foreword

Since the advent of stoma nursing over 30 years ago, the development of nursing roles in gastroenterology clinical practice has widened significantly. This book explores the fundamental aspects of nursing patients who have gastrointestinal problems. It is targeted primarily toward the student nurse or the nurse who is preparing to work for the first time in a clinical area that manages gastrointestinal problems. Clinical nursing practice is advancing, and a key element of skilled clinical practice is advocacy. Today's nurses can now broaden their ability to advocate for the needs of patients with gastrointestinal problems: essential skills, given the stigma and embarrassment that surround many of these problems.

Each chapter provides the nurse with a clear description of the gastrointestinal disease, the assessment and diagnostic pathway of the patient and a practical and clear delineation of the clinical skills and knowledge required to care holistically for the patient. The book brings together an impressive group of academics and clinical practitioners, all experts in their field, to create a practical and relevant text. After reading this book nurses will have advanced their knowledge in this field of nursing and will be assured that the care they provide is appropriately prioritised and built around the needs of the patient. This is the first book of its kind – it fills an educational gap and is sure to inform, inspire and motivate the future generation of clinical nurse specialists in gastroenterology.

Theresa Porrett, PhD, MSc, RN
Gastrointestinal Nurse Consultant, Homerton University Hospital NHS
Foundation Trust, London
Honorary Reader, Department of Applied Biological Sciences, City
University, London

Preface

This text has been written for the student nurse and aspiring gastrointestinal nurse who wishes to launch their career in gastrointestinal practice as well as for nurses who want to inform their thinking about gastrointestinal disorders and their nursing management. Throughout, perspectives on practice emerge that will promote the formation of new thinking in relation to the fundamental aspects of gastrointestinal nursing. In each chapter aspects of practice are presented to assist in the development, implementation and evaluation of gastrointestinal nursing practice.

In Chapter 1 the foundation for considering nursing care associated with a variety of gastrointestinal disorders is described. It reflects on the context in which care is provided and the professional role of the nurse. It provides a viewpoint on accountability and managing risk associated with the complexities of gastrointestinal nursing and concludes by acknowledging that gastrointestinal nursing does not exist in isolation. It exists within an environment in which it is integral to, and forms an essential part of, the multidisciplinary team responsible for the care of patients who have gastrointestinal disease and disorders.

Chapter 2 articulates the anatomy and physiology of the gastrointestinal tract. It provides background knowledge for the chapters that follow so that the aspiring nurse as well as the practising nurse or allied health professional can understand the complexities of diseases and disorders within the practice of gastrointestinal care.

Chapter 3 discusses nutrition, including the components of a healthy diet. It indicates that constituents such as proteins, lipids, carbohydrates, minerals and vitamins are essential elements that should be balanced in a healthy diet. Malnutrition, dehydration, screening and assessment of nutritional status, food poisoning and its causes and prevention are discussed. Consideration is also given to the issues of food poverty, food security and the politics of food.

Chapter 4 relates to complaints of the upper gastrointestinal tract. Conditions of the oesophagus, stomach and duodenum, and cancer of the upper gastrointestinal tract are discussed. At the conclusion of the chapter knowledge of the various upper gastrointestinal complaints will be improved. By reading the chapter, student and practising nurses will have a greater understanding of the management options available and the diagnostic tests that patients with upper gastrointestinal symptoms may undergo. Finally, the lifestyle changes that some patients with upper gastrointestinal complaints may find beneficial are presented.

Chapter 5 involves consideration of constipation, diarrhoea, wind and bloating, rectal pain and bleeding, mesenteric ischaemia, perforation, appendicitis, occult gastrointestinal (GI) bleeding, intestinal obstruction, intra-abdominal abscesses and pancreatitis. Each condition is defined in association with its epidemiology and pathophysiology. Its assessment, diagnosis and associated care planning with nursing interventions are also discussed. At the conclusion of the chapter, key points are presented to assist the student or practising nurse in caring for patients with lower GI complaints.

Chapter 6 reflects on tumours of the gastrointestinal tract. The epidemiology, pathophysiology, aetiology, signs and symptoms, diagnosis and management of gastrointestinal tumours provide the background for the provision of nursing care. The nursing process, including diagnosis and care planning as well as implementation of various interventions, are discussed to assist the student and practising nurse in the provision of care to patients with gastrointestinal tumours.

Chapter 7 addresses malabsorption syndrome. It is indicated that malabsorption is not a diagnosis but a range of syndromes that occur when nutrients are not absorbed from within the gastrointestinal tract. Pathophysiology, including inflammation and infection, structural abnormalities, insufficient digestive agents and impaired transport, forms the foundation knowledge for appropriate nursing care. Assessment, diagnosis, care planning and nursing interventions conclude the chapter to assist the student or practising nurse or allied health professional in the provision of care.

Chapter 8 explores the chronic disorder of inflammatory bowel disease, which typically presents in early adulthood. It provides a fundamental understanding of inflammatory bowel disease that will enable the student or practising nurse to assess, plan and deliver immediate care for this patient group. It also focuses on the long-term support required for the person with a chronic debilitating illness.

Chapter 9 considers a range of procedures used in imaging of the gastrointestinal tract. It gives a brief description of each procedure, along with patient preparation and aftercare. It is noted that the gastrointestinal tract can be difficult to image well, as it does not show up clearly on images. Various factors considering this conundrum are discussed. The use of contrast agents and good bowel preparation are described to show how much of this problem can be overcome.

Chapter 10 explores a range of conditions that cannot be neatly categorised as arising within a part of the gastrointestinal tract, but for which they have significant implications. Diseases addressed include coeliac disease, anorexia nervosa, reactive arthritis, gastrointestinal anthrax and trichinosis. Epidemiology, pathophysiology, assessment, diagnosis and treatment, including the provision of nursing care, are described in association with each disease.

The authors who have contributed to this book are experts in the field of gastrointestinal nursing practice. They have written each chapter with the intention of providing knowledge that will promote skill development in gastrointestinal nursing practice. We think you will enjoy reading this text.

Carol L. Cox, Martin J. Steggall and Alison M. Coutts

Acknowledgement

Special thanks are expressed to Mariann Baulf for her advisory capacity in Chapter 10: Other diseases.

Contributors

Daniel Apau, MSc, BSc, ENB 100, RGN
Lecturer, Advanced Practice, School of Health Sciences, City University London
(Chapter 6)

Warren Chapman, MSc Advanced Practice (Nursing), RN
JAG accredited upper and lower GI Endoscopist
Nurse Consultant, Endoscopy Unit, City Hospital, Sandwell and West Birmingham
Hospitals NHS Trust, Birmingham
(Chapters 4 and 10)

Alison M. Coutts, MSc, BSc, PGCEA, RGN
Senior Lecturer Applied Biological Sciences, School of Health Sciences, City
University London
(Chapters 3 and 7)

Carol L. Cox, PhD, MSc, MA Ed, PG Dip Ed, BSc (Hons), RN, FHEA
Professor of Nursing, Advanced Clinical Practice, Department of Applied
Biological Sciences, School of Health Sciences, City University London
(Chapters 1 and 5)

Jennifer C. Edie, MEd, TDCR, DMU
Senior Lecturer, Radiography, School of Health Sciences, City University London
(Chapter 9)

Martin J. Steggall, PhD, MSc, BSc (Hons), RN (Adult), FHEA
Associate Dean, Pre-registration Undergraduate Nursing and Midwifery, School
of Health Sciences, City University London
(Chapter 2)

Julia Williams, MEd, BSc (Hons), Dip D/N, RGN
Senior Lecturer Burdett Institute of Gastrointestinal Nursing, Burdett Institute of Gastrointestinal Nursing with King's College and St. Mark's Hospital, Harrow, London
    (Chapter 8)

CHAPTER 1

Introduction to the fundamental aspects of gastrointestinal nursing

Carol L. Cox

Introduction

The practice of gastrointestinal nursing is both a science and an art. It requires specialised knowledge and skills to provide holistic care to patients and to ensure positive patient experiences in both health and illness. Practice as a gastrointestinal nurse occurs in a variety of environments. Gastrointestinal nurses may find themselves practising in an outpatient clinic, ward or palliative care unit as well as working in patients' homes as nurse specialists. The purpose of this book is to articulate the fundamental aspects of nursing patients who have gastrointestinal disorders. It is targeted primarily toward the student nurse or nurse who is preparing to work in a clinical environment that manages gastrointestinal disorders for the first time. However, it also has specific relevance for practice nurses working in general practice surgeries and district and health visiting nurses who need to recognise gastrointestinal disorders when managing their patient caseloads. It also has relevance for allied health professionals practising within primary and secondary care who wish to gain fundamental knowledge about gastrointestinal disorders.

Providing holistic care to patients with gastrointestinal disorders requires an understanding of basic human needs and the ability to grasp patients' understanding of their health and illness within the context of their cultural background. Nursing theories and models of care and models like the Health Belief Model (Becker, 1974) are essential knowledge that impart a basis and rationale for practice. They also render a focus for nursing care. The patient's physical, intellectual, psychosocial, cultural, ethnic, spiritual and environmental factors must all be taken into account when promoting wellness, preventing illness and fostering the development of coping mechanisms (Watson, 1999, 2008). In addition, an understanding of the attitudes and values that influence human behaviour and the ethical dimensions of nursing practice (Nursing and Midwifery Council (NMC), 2008) are essential components of the nurse's toolkit in the management of patient care.

Activity
Reflect on the models of care that you have learned about as a student at university. Which ones have influenced your world view about practice?

This chapter establishes the foundation for considering nursing care associated with a variety of gastrointestinal disorders. It considers the context in which care is provided and the professional role of the nurse. It provides a viewpoint on accountability and managing risk associated with the complexities of gastrointestinal nursing and concludes by acknowledging that gastrointestinal nursing does not exist in isolation. Gastrointestinal nursing has broadened within all areas of its specialism and exists within an environment in which it is integral and forms an essential part of the multidisciplinary team responsible for the care of patients that have gastrointestinal diseases and disorders.

Context of care and professionalism
The context in which nursing care is provided is undergoing significant change in the National Health Service (NHS) and throughout the global health economy (Cox, 2011; Cox and Hall, 2007). The changing context requires an entirely new level of professionalism. Professionalism can be defined as 'the conduct, aims, or qualities that characterise or mark a profession or a professional person' (Merriam-Webster, 2003, p. 991). In assuming the professional role, the nurse conforms to the technical and ethical standards of nursing, exhibiting a courteous, conscientious and generally businesslike manner in the workplace (NMC, 2008). Within the context of a busy clinic or ward maintaining such behaviour can be fraught with difficulties. It requires having a cool head when it may appear everyone about the nurse is losing theirs.

According to Brehm *et al.* (2006) the concept of professionalism is multifaceted. Professionalism may be divided into three components or categories: professional parameters, professional behaviours and professional responsibilities (Bossers *et al.*, 1999). Professional parameters include legal and ethical issues, whilst professional behaviours are related to discipline-related knowledge and skills: relationships with patients and colleagues in which collaboration and collegiality become essential components and an acceptable appearance and attitude. Professional responsibilities relate to a responsibility to the nursing profession, to oneself, patients, employers and the community. Nurses must develop the full spectrum of characteristics, attitudes and behaviours, including a lifelong commitment to professionalism if they are to be regarded as a professional.

Activity
Describe what the Nursing and Midwifery Council states in the code (NMC, 2008) regarding confidentiality, collaboration, professional boundaries and acting with integrity.

Accountability and managing risk

Part of professionalism is being accountable for interventions undertaken by the nurse. Gastrointestinal diseases and disorders require a variety of interventions that can lead to serious consequences for patients when the organisation in which the nurse works has not put in place the correct systems and processes to prevent incidents from happening, when procedures have not been followed (generally due to poor observation) or when a nurse disregards protocol (generally due to lack of judgement). Serious untoward incidents (also known as SUIs) are now termed 'never events' by the Department of Health (DoH, 2011a):

> 'Never events' are very serious, largely preventable patient safety incidents that should not occur if the relevant preventative measures have been put in place. (DoH, 2011a, p. 1)

Gastrointestinal nurses should know that for an incident to be identified as a 'never event' it must fulfil the following criteria:

- The incident has clear potential for or has caused severe harm/death.

- There is evidence of occurrence in the past (i.e. it is a known source of risk).

- There is existing national guidance and/or national safety recommendations on how the event can be prevented and support for implementation.

- The event is largely preventable if the guidance is implemented.

- Occurrence can be easily defined, identified and continually measured (DoH, 2011b, p. 4).

Examples of various types of incident that can occur include: perforation of the oesophagus during endoscopic dilatation of oesophageal strictures; excessive restriction of the stomach during bariatric surgery; poor siting of a stoma; theft of prescription forms (FP10s); delays of biopsy results; and lost referral of patients who have been diagnosed with gastrointestinal tumours.

The Department of Health (DoH, 2011b) has published 25 'never events' that should be regarded as unacceptable in the health service. These are:

1. Wrong site surgery (existing)
2. Wrong implant/prosthesis (new)
3. Retained foreign object post-operation (existing)
4. Wrongly prepared high-risk injectable medication (new)
5. Maladministration of potassium-containing solutions (modified)
6. Wrong route administration of chemotherapy (existing)
7. Wrong route administration of oral/enteral treatment (new)
8. Intravenous administration of epidural medication (new)
9. Maladministration of insulin (new)
10. Overdose of midazolam during conscious sedation (new)
11. Opioid overdose of an opioid-naïve patient (new)
12. Inappropriate administration of daily oral methotrexate (new)
13. Suicide using non-collapsible rails (existing)
14. Escape of a transferred prisoner (existing)
15. Falls from unrestricted windows (new)
16. Entrapment in bedrails (new)
17. Transfusion of ABO-incompatible blood components (new)
18. Transplantation of ABO or HLA-incompatible organs (new)
19. Misplaced naso- or orogastric tubes (modified)
20. Wrong gas administered (new)
21. Failure to monitor and respond to oxygen saturation (new)
22. Air embolism (new)
23. Misidentification of patients (new)
24. Severe scalding of patients (new)
25. Maternal death due to post partum haemorrhage after elective Caesarean section (modified)

(DoH, 2011, pp. 18–32)

This list of incidents should not be regarded as the sum total of serious incidents. Incidents occurring outside of this list would also be considered as 'serious'. Therefore gastrointestinal nurses must be continually cognisant of the element of risk (Taylor and Watson, 1989).

Activity
Articulate what the Nursing and Midwifery Council states in the code (NMC, 2008) regarding managing risk.

Emslie (2002) has indicated that the issue of managing risk is more important today than in the past, as healthcare provision has become more complex. In order to manage risk, the causes and types of errors that can lead to 'never events' must be identified. Identification should be within the healthcare organisation itself and within the context of the nurse's individual practice. The types of error that can occur are (Roberts, 2002):

■ Type I – Omission
■ Type II – Commission
■ Type III – Unawareness

Omission typically involves a 'failure to comply with current regulations or statute or to fail to comply with current professionally accepted practice' (Roberts, 2002, p. 17). This may be due to a nurse's lack of knowledge, which could be associated with inadequate training or failure to engage in learning activities that keep knowledge up to date.

Commission is any act committed that should not have been. Roberts (2002, p. 17) indicates that commission is associated with a 'lack of commitment or consideration for others involved in the healthcare process'. For example, a gastrointestinal nurse specialist may be performing an endoscopy and perforate the bowel whilst taking a sample for biopsy. This results in serious injury to the patient. St John Holt (2011) indicates that there is a moral objective in accident prevention whereby there is a duty of reasonable care owed to others.

Unawareness arises from 'a faulty specification of the nature of a problem which leads to real solutions being adopted to deal with wrongly identified problems, rather than incorrect solutions to real problems' (Roberts, 2002, p. 18). In this case errors occur through a lack of understanding about what the real problem is, or assumptions are made about what the problem might be. This type of error is most frequently associated with management decisions. Managers can become out of touch with practice; they are not fully aware of what is occurring in the clinical setting for which they are responsible and can make decisions that impact on service delivery, resulting in potential harm to patients and staff alike (Hoffman and Perry, 2005).

The government has indicated (DoH, 2011b, p. 7) that:

> In the real world we accept that there is the possibility that unforeseen scenarios could mean that a 'never event' may not have been preventable... and that in individual cases, (where) it can be shown that completely unanticipated or unpreventable circumstances led to an event occurring, we would suggest the commissioner and provider should agree not to classify it as a 'never event'

In relation to the gastrointestinal nurse's responsibility for managing risk, it is crucial that issues are considered and discussed before serious incidents occur in the healthcare environment to ensure that prevention strategies are implemented. This is an essential principle in managing risk.

It is the responsibility of every practising gastrointestinal nurse to develop their professional knowledge, skills and behaviours beyond that which they were assessed against for entry to the professional register (CHRE, 2009; NMC, 2008). This equates to ongoing professional development through continuing education initiatives. Robust and well-managed risk management processes are the foundation upon which patients are protected against 'never events'.

Activity
Explain what the Nursing and Midwifery Council means in the code (NMC, 2008) about keeping your skills and knowledge up to date.

Summary
This chapter has established the foundation for considering nursing care associated with a variety of gastrointestinal disorders. It considers the context in which care is provided and the professional role of the nurse. It provides a viewpoint on accountability and managing risk associated with the complexities of gastrointestinal nursing and concludes by acknowledging that gastrointestinal nursing does not exist in isolation. Gastrointestinal nursing has broadened within all areas of its specialism and exists within an environment in which it is integral

and forms an essential part of the multidisciplinary team responsible for the care of patients that have gastrointestinal disease and disorders.

References

Becker, M. (1974) The health belief model and personal health behavior. *Health Education Monographs*, **2**, 324–473.

Bossers, A., Kernaghan, J., Hodgins, L., Merla, L., O'Connor, C. and Van Kessel, M. (1999) Defining and developing professionalism. *Canadian Journal of Occupational Therapy*, **66**(3), 16–21.

Brehm, B., Breen, P., Brown, B., Long, L., Smith, R., Wall, A. and Warren, N. (2006) Instructional design and assessment: an interdisciplinary approach to introducing professionalism. *American Journal of Pharmaceutical Education*, **70**(4), 1–5.

CHRE (2009) *Advanced Practice: Report to the Four UK Health Departments*. Council for Healthcare Regulatory Excellence, Peterborough.

Cox, C. (2011) Professionalism in advanced practice: the professional role. In: *Advanced Practice in Healthcare: Skills for Nurses and Allied Health Professionals* (eds. C. Cox, M. Hill and V. Lack). Routledge, Abingdon.

Cox, C. and Hall, A. (2007) Advanced practice role in gastrointestinal nursing. *Journal of Gastrointestinal Nursing*, **5**(4), 26–31.

Department of Health (2011a) *Patient Safety*. http://www.dh.gov.uk/en/Healthcare/Patient-safety/index.htm (accessed 28 August 2011).

Department of Health (2011b) *Never Events List 2011/2012: Policy Framework for use in the NHS*. http://www.dh.gov.uk/en/Publicationsandstatistics/Publications/index.htm (accessed 28 August 2011).

Emslie, S. (2002) Foreword. In: *Risk Management in Healthcare*, 2nd edn (ed. G. Roberts). Witherby & Co., London.

Hoffman, P. and Perry, F. (2005) *Management Mistakes in Healthcare*. Cambridge Press, New York.

Merriam-Webster's Collegiate Dictionary (2003) *Merriam-Webster's Collegiate Dictionary*, 11th edn. Merriam-Webster, Springfield, MA.

Nursing and Midwifery Council (NMC) (2008) *The Code: Standards of Conduct, Performance and Ethics for Nurses and Midwives*. Nursing and Midwifery Council, London.

Roberts, G. (2002) *Risk Management in Healthcare*, 2nd edn. Witherby & Co., London.

St John Holt, A. (2011) *Principles of Health and Safety at Work*, 8th edn. Lavenham Press, IOSH Services, Leicester.

Taylor, R. and Watson, J. (eds.) (1989) *They Shall not Hurt: Human Suffering and Human Caring*. University Press of Colorado, Boulder.

Watson, J. (1999) *Post Modern Nursing and Beyond.* Churchill Livingstone, London.

Watson, J. (2008) *Nursing. The Philosophy and Science of Caring*, rev. edn. Boulder: University Press of Colorado

CHAPTER 2

Anatomy and physiology of the gastrointestinal system

Martin Steggall

Introduction

In this chapter an overview of the anatomy and physiology of the gastrointestinal (GI) system will be considered. The main functions of the GI system involve:

- Ingestion of raw materials
- The breakdown or digestion (physically and chemically) of the raw material into smaller particles
- Absorption of those particles into the bloodstream
- Elimination of waste or unusable material

By reading this chapter and carrying out the proposed activities you should achieve the following learning outcomes:

- Improve your knowledge of the anatomy and physiology of the GI system
- Understand the processes of ingestion, mastication, digestion, secretion, absorption and excretion (defecation)
- Discuss hormones associated with the digestive process

The digestive tract (or alimentary canal), is a muscular tube that contains the organs of the digestive system (Figure 2.1). This tube begins at the mouth and ends at the anus. Between these two points are the pharynx, oesophagus, stomach, and small and large intestines. In addition, accessory organs (such as teeth, salivary glands, liver, pancreas and gallbladder) are necessary for processing materials into usable substances.

The components of the digestive system work together to perform the following general steps:

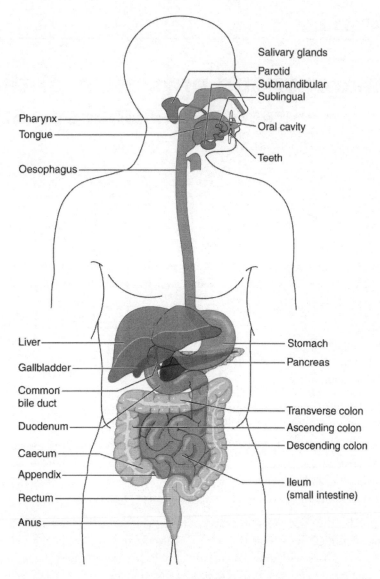

Figure 2.1 The digestive system.

1. Ingestion
2. Mastication
3. Digestion

4. Secretion
5. Absorption
6. Excretion (defecation)

Initially food enters the mouth, an activity called ingestion. Once food is ingested, the tongue and teeth work together to mechanically process the food by physically breaking it down. The chewing action is called mastication. Digestion is the chemical process of breaking down food into small molecules, which is necessary so that nutrients can be absorbed by the lining of the digestive tract. The secretion of acids, buffers, enzymes and water aid in the breakdown of food. Once the food is broken down, both physically and chemically, it is ready for absorption through the lining of the digestive tract for use by the body. Finally, waste products and unusable materials are prepared for excretion and are eliminated by the body through defecation.

Organs of the alimentary canal

Mouth
Food enters the digestive tract through the mouth or buccal cavity. The lips or labia protect the opening of the buccal cavity. There are *hard* and *soft* palates that create the roof of the chamber, while the tongue acts as the floor (Figure 2.2). The tongue's base and the uvula (the finger-like projection at the back of the mouth), are the boundary between the oral cavity and the next part of the digestive system, the pharynx. The sides of the cavity are created by the cheeks. The mouth and oral cavity region receive, or *ingest*, food. The food is tasted, *mechanically* broken down into smaller pieces, and *chemically* broken down to some degree. Liquid is added to make it easier to swallow.

Tongue
The tongue is a muscle that provides taste stimuli to the brain, senses temperature and texture (as does the rest of the mouth), manipulates food while chewing and aids in swallowing. As the tongue moves food around in the oral cavity, saliva is added to moisten and soften food, while teeth continue to crush the food until it reaches the right consistency. The tongue pushes the food into a ball-like mass called a bolus so that it can be passed on to the pharynx. A membrane under the tongue, called the lingual frenulum, which can be seen when the tongue is lifted, prevents the tongue from being swallowed. The tongue helps prepare the bolus of food, then the tip of the tongue lifts up and the bolus moves to the back of the mouth, coming into contact with the soft palate. All of these processes are

11

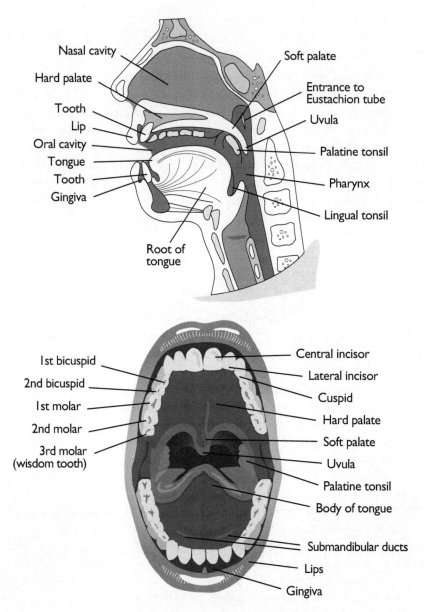

Figure 2.2 The mouth and oral cavity.

under voluntary control, but as soon as the bolus comes into contact with the soft palate, the process comes under autonomic control. The remainder of the digestive process remains under autonomic control.

Taste

In order to taste food, it must be in solution. Dry foods have no taste. Taste occurs because of the presence of taste papillae, comprising of several taste buds. These occur throughout the mucous membranes of the mouth, tongue, pharynx and upper oesophagus. There are five different types of taste buds: bitter, sweet, sour, salty and umami. Additionally, and perhaps controversially, water is thought to be a recognisable taste. Umami is the most recently identified, and is a savoury, meaty taste.

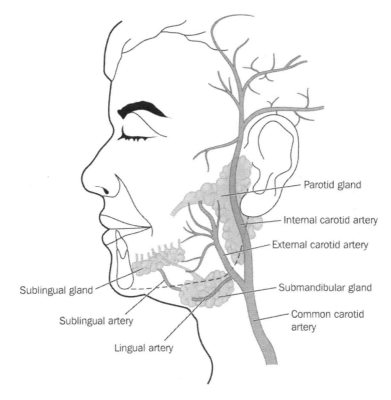

Figure 2.3 The salivary glands.

Salivary glands

As can be seen in Figure 2.3, there are three pairs of salivary glands, which are controlled by the autonomic nervous system. A large parotid salivary gland is found slightly inferior and anterior to each ear. The ducts from these glands empty into the upper portion of the oral cavity. The smallest of the salivary glands, the sublingual salivary glands, are located under the tongue. The submandibular salivary glands are located on both sides along the inner surfaces of the mandible, or lower jaw.

On average, these glands collectively produce *1–1.5 litres of saliva daily*. Small amounts of saliva are continuously produced to keep the mouth moist, but once eating or even thinking about eating begins, saliva is formed in greater quantities. Saliva is almost totally water (99.4%) but it also contains some antibodies, buffers, ions, waste products and enzymes. Enzymes are organic catalysts that speed up chemical reactions. Salivary amylase is one of the digestive enzymes that breaks down carbohydrates, such as starches, into smaller molecules, such as glucose, that are more easily absorbed by the digestive tract once they get there. Saliva also cleans the oral surfaces and aids in reducing the quantity of bacteria that grow in the mouth.

Activity

Older people frequently suffer from xerostoma from salivary gland malfunction (Turner and Ship, 2007; Ship *et al.*, 2002). This means they have 'dry mouths'. This makes it more difficult for them to moisten food. Describe the actions you can undertake to moisten older patients' mouths so that it is easier for them to eat.

Teeth

The final important components of the mechanical aspect of digestion in the oral cavity are the teeth. The first set of teeth are called deciduous teeth, as they are not permanent. They begin to appear at around 6 months of age, the first being the lower central incisors, with all 20 usually in place by 2 years of age. Between the ages of 6 and 12 years these teeth are pushed out and replaced by the 32 larger *permanent teeth*. The exceptions to this are the *wisdom teeth*, which may not appear until an individual is as old as 21 years.

Pharynx

The pharynx is a common passageway not only for food and water but also for air. It has three parts: the *nasopharynx*, the *oropharynx* and the *laryngopharynx*. The nasopharynx is primarily part of the respiratory system. The oropharynx and the laryngopharynx serve as a passageway for food and water and for air. During swallowing, it is imperative that the passageways to the nasal and respiratory regions are protected from the accidental introduction of food and liquids. The nasopharynx is blocked by the soft palate, and a flap of tissue called the epiglottis covers the airway to the lungs as the trachea rises during swallowing. These actions force the food to enter the only possible route, which is the oesophagus.

Oesophagus

The oesophagus is approximately 25 centimetres long and is responsible for transporting food from the pharynx to the stomach. It extends from the pharynx, through the thoracic cavity and diaphragm, to the stomach, which is located in the peritoneal cavity (Figure 2.4).

The oesophagus is normally a collapsed tube until a bolus of food is swallowed. As this bolus moves to the oesophagus, a muscular ring at the beginning of this structure, called the pharyngo-oesophageal sphincter, relaxes. The muscles of the oesophagus begin rhythmic contractions that move the food down to the stomach. This rhythmic muscular contraction is known as peristalsis. Once the bolus reaches the end of the oesophagus, the lower oesophageal sphincter (which used to be called the *cardiac sphincter*) relaxes to let food into the stomach. The sphincter then closes to prevent acidic gastric juices from entering the oesophagus.

The oesophagus also helps move the bolus by secreting mucus so that its walls are slippery. The oesophageal walls are lined with stratified squamous epithelium, which makes the oesophagus resistant to abrasion, temperature extremes and irritation by chemicals.

Walls of the alimentary canal

The same four basic tissue types form the wall of the entire alimentary canal from the oesophagus onward (Figure 2.5). The innermost layer that lines the lumen of the canal is the mucosa. This layer is composed mostly of surface epithelium with some connective tissue and a thin smooth muscle layer surrounding it. The mucosa also possesses cells that secrete *digestive enzymes* to break down foodstuffs, and *goblet cells* that secrete *mucus* for lubrication.

The submucosa is the next layer and is composed of soft connective tissue. This layer contains blood and lymph vessels, lymph nodes (called Peyer's patches,

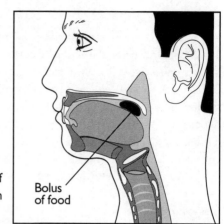

Figure 2.4 Movement of a bolus of food from the mouth to the stomach via the oesophagus.

Bolus of food

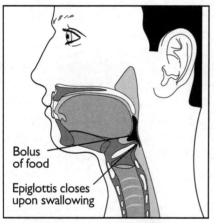

Bolus of food

Epiglottis closes upon swallowing

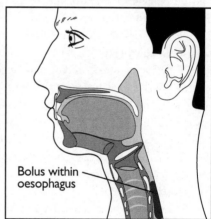

Bolus within oesophagus

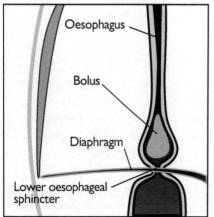

Oesophagus

Bolus

Diaphragm

Lower oesophageal sphincter

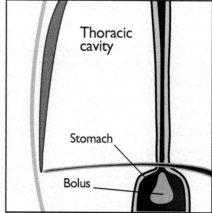

Thoracic cavity

Stomach

Bolus

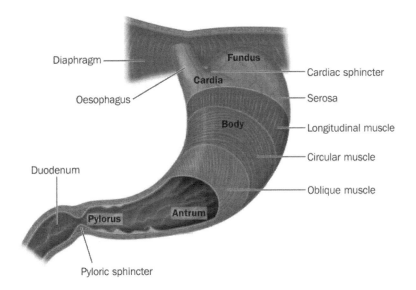

Figure 2.5 Basic tissue types of the alimentary canal.

which are similar to the tonsils), and nerve endings. The next layer is the muscularis externa, which is composed of two layers of smooth muscle.

The outermost layer is the serosa, composed of a single thin layer of flat, serous, fluid-producing cells supported by connective tissue. For most of the canal, the serosa is the *visceral peritoneum*. The peritoneum is a serous membrane in the abdominopelvic cavity. Like all serous membranes it has two layers. The visceral peritoneum covers the organs and the parietal peritoneum lines the wall of the abdominopelvic cavity. Between the layers is a fluid-filled potential space called the peritoneal cavity. This fluid is important for both keeping the outer surface of the intestines moist and allowing friction-free movement of the digestive organs against the abdominopelvic cavity. Some abdominal organs such as the urinary bladder and the duodenum are not surrounded by peritoneum and are called retroperitoneal organs. The oesophagus differs in that it possesses only a loose layer of connective tissue called the adventitia.

Stomach

The stomach is located in the left side of the abdominal cavity under the diaphragm and is covered almost completely by the liver. This organ is approximately 25 cm long with a diameter that varies, depending on how much food is taken at any given time. Although the stomach can hold up to 4 litres when totally filled, it can expand or decrease in diameter thanks to deep folds, called rugae (singular rugus), in the stomach wall that allow for these size changes. As the stomach receives food from the oesophagus, it performs several functions:

- Acts as a temporary holding area for the received food
- Secretes gastric acid and enzymes, which it mixes with the food, causing chemical digestion
- Regulates the rate at which the now partially digested food (a thick, heavy, creamlike liquid called chyme) enters the small intestine
- Absorbs small amounts of water and substances on a very limited basis (although the stomach does absorb alcohol)

On average it takes between 4 and 6 hours for the stomach to empty after a meal. Liquids and carbohydrates pass through in about 4 hours. Protein takes a little more time, and fats take longer, usually about 6 hours.

The stomach is divided into four regions. Located near the heart, the *cardiac region* surrounds the lower oesophageal sphincter (Figure 2.6). The fundus, which is actually lateral and slightly superior to the cardiac region, temporarily holds the food when it initially enters the stomach. The *body* is the mid-portion and largest region of the stomach. The funnel-shaped terminal end of the stomach is called the pylorus. Most of the digestive work of the stomach is performed in the pyloric

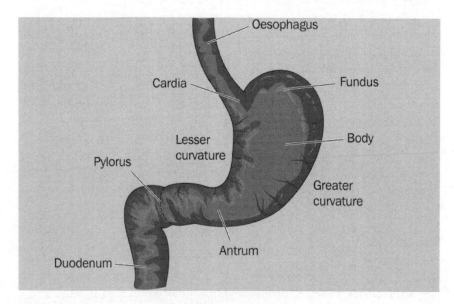

Figure 2.6 The stomach.

region. This is also the region where chyme must pass through another opening, the pyloric sphincter, in order to enter the small intestine.

The muscular action of the stomach works much like a cement mixer and is achieved by the three layers of muscle found in its walls. One layer is *longitudinal*, one is *circular* and the third is *oblique* in orientation. This arrangement of muscles enables the stomach to churn food as it mixes with gastric juices excreted by *gastric glands* from *gastric pits* in the columnar epithelial lining of the stomach as well as to work the food toward the pyloric sphincter through muscle activity termed peristalsis. With the combined efforts of muscle and gastric juices, both physical and chemical digestion occur in the stomach.

Gastric juice is a general term for a combination of *hydrochloric acid* (HCl), *pepsinogen* and *mucus*. About 1500 millilitres of gastric juice is produced each day by gastric glands. Pepsinogen is secreted by the *chief cells*; it is the inactive precursor to pepsin, the stomach's main digestive enzyme. HCl is secreted by *parietal cells*. These two cell types have a special relationship: it is HCl that promotes the conversion of pepsinogen to pepsin. Pepsin is needed to break down proteins (like the ones found in meat). The stomachs of children also release rennin, which facilitates protein digestion, particularly milk protein. HCl doesn't directly digest food, but it breaks down connective tissue in meat. HCl is a strong acid, with a pH of around 1.5 to 2. This highly acidic environment also aids in destroying pathogens that might enter the stomach. The stomach is protected from HCl by *mucous cells* that generate a thick layer of mucus, which then shields the stomach lining from the effects of HCl. In addition, pepsinogen is not converted to pepsin until it comes into contact with HCl, which does not occur until it is safely within the lumen of the stomach, away from the mucosal walls. Other specialised cells secrete what is known as *intrinsic factor*, which is needed for absorption of vitamin B$_{12}$ (Table 2.1).

Table 2.1 Gastric glands and their functions.

Digestive cells	Secretion type	Function
Chief cells	Pepsinogen	Begins digestion of protein
Parietal cells	HCl	Kills pathogens; activates pepsinogen, which is converted to pepsin; breaks down connective tissue in meat
Mucous cells	Alkaline mucus	Protects stomach lining
Endocrine cells	Gastrin	Stimulates gastric gland secretion

The stomach's activity is controlled by the parasympathetic nervous system, particularly the *vagus nerve*. Once the vagus nerve is stimulated, the stomach's *motility* (churning action) increases, as do the secretory rates of the gastric glands.

Activity

Some patients undergo a surgical procedure called bariatric surgery so that they can lose weight. Review information about bariatric surgery and its implications for nursing care in Apau and Whiteing's (2011) article published in the *Journal of Gastrointestinal Nursing*.

Small intestine

Located in the central and lower abdominal cavity, the small intestine is, surprisingly, *the* major organ of digestion. It is where most food is digested (Figure 2.7). The small intestine is small in diameter, not in length. Beginning at the pyloric sphincter, the small intestine is also the longest section of the alimentary canal, with a length of up to 6 metres and a diameter ranging from 4 centimetres where it connects with the stomach to 2.5 centimetres where it meets the large intestine.

The pancreas empties into the small intestine at the first curvature of the duodenum. Pancreatic juice includes most of the enzymes required for the initial

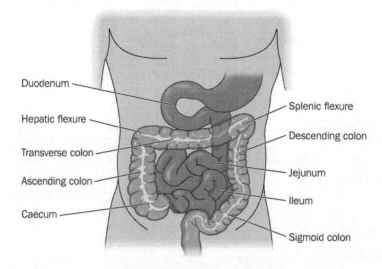

Figure 2.7 The intestines.

stages of digestion, so digestion will occur throughout the small intestine, although as the material progresses, digestion is completed and absorption becomes more important. The walls of the small intestine secrete several digestive enzymes important for the final stages of chemical digestion and two hormones that stimulate the pancreas and gallbladder to act and control stomach activity.

In the small intestine, almost 80% of the absorption of usable nutrients takes place when chyme comes into contact with the mucosal walls. Amino acids, fatty acids, ions, simple sugars, vitamins and water are all absorbed here. Some of the remaining 20% has already been absorbed by the stomach, with the rest being absorbed by the large intestine. Any residue that cannot be utilised is sent on to the large intestine for removal from the body.

There are three regions of the small intestine. The duodenum is approximately 25 centimetres long and is located near the head of the pancreas. The jejunum is the middle section and is approximately 2.5 metres long. The terminal end of the small intestine is the ileum. This 2 metre section attaches to the large intestine at the *ileocaecal valve*.

The pyloric sphincter is important in allowing small portions of chyme to enter the first part of the small intestine (duodenum) because the small intestine can process only small amounts of food at a time. At the duodenum, additional secretions are added from the pancreas and gallbladder. The pancreas provides pancreatic juices and the gallbladder provides bile. Bile *emulsifies* fat; that is, it makes fat able to disperse in water. Pancreatic juice contains enzymes and sodium bicarbonate, which neutralise the acidic chyme. The pancreas is stimulated to secrete as a result of the hormone *secretin*, which is produced by the small intestine. Gallbladder activity is caused by the hormone cholecystokinin, also known as CCK, which is also produced by the small intestine. Two types of muscular action occur in the small intestine. Segmentation is the muscle action that mixes chyme and digestive juices, working much like a cement mixer. Peristalsis also occurs, moving undigested food remains toward the large intestine. Refer to Table 2.2 for the hormones active in the digestive process.

The small intestine also produces digestive enzymes that are needed to complete chemical digestion. These enzymes (and mucus) are produced by exocrine cells. *Lactase, maltase* and *sucrase* are needed for the digestion of double sugars called *disaccharides* that are contained in starches. *Peptidase* is needed to digest small proteins called peptides. Internal *lipase* is needed for digestion of certain fats. The acidity of chyme results in chemical and mechanical irritation, which distends or stretches the intestinal walls, resulting in the release of the enzymes and the two hormones.

Table 2.2 Hormones in the digestive process.

Hormone	Secreting organ	Action
Gastrin	Stomach	Stimulates release of gastric juice
Secretin	Duodenum	Stimulates release of bicarbonate and water from the pancreas and bile from the liver; slows stomach activity
Cholecystokinin (CCK)	Duodenum	Stimulates digestive enzyme release from the pancreas and bile release from the gallbladder; slows stomach activity

The wall of the small intestine contains circular folds called *plicae circulares* and finger-like protrusions into the lumen called villi (Figure 2.8). The villi also have outer layers of columnar epithelial cells, which possess microscopic extensions known as *microvilli*. These villi are tightly packed, giving a velvety texture and appearance. The purpose of the microvilli, villi and circular folds is to

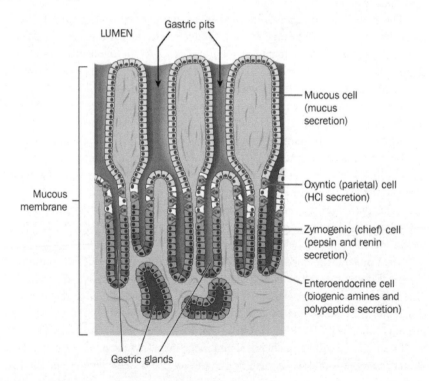

Figure 2.8 Villi.

provide an incredible increase in the surface area of the small intestine, increasing the efficiency of the absorption of nutrients.

Each villus contains a network of capillaries and a lymphatic capillary called a lacteal. Intestinal glands are located between villi. The capillaries absorb and transport sugars (the result of carbohydrate digestion) and amino acids (the result of protein digestion) to the liver for further processing before they are sent throughout the body. Glycerol and fatty acids (obtained from the digestion of fat) are absorbed by the villi and converted into a lipoprotein that travels on to the lacteal, where it becomes a white, milky substance called chyle. Chyle goes directly into the lymphatic system for distribution throughout the body.

> **Activity**
> Some patients have coeliac disease – refer to Chapter 10 for information about this disease. Consider the nursing implications for a patient who suffers from damage to the lining of the small intestine.

Large intestine

Beginning at the junction with the end of the small intestine (*ileocaecal orifice*) and extending to the anus, the large intestine almost totally borders the small intestine (Figure 2.9). The large intestine is responsible for:

- Water reabsorption
- Absorption of vitamins produced by normal bacteria in the large intestine
- Packaging and compacting waste products for elimination from the body

Since there are no villi in the walls of the large intestine, little nutrient absorption occurs here.

Approximately 1.5 metres long and 6 centimetres in diameter, the large intestine is divided into three main regions: the caecum, colon and rectum.

The caecum, a pouch-shaped structure, receives any undigested food (such as cellulose) and water from the ileum of the small intestine. The appendix is attached to the caecum. About 9 centimetres long, the appendix is a slender, hollow, dead-end tube lined with lymphatic tissue. Since it is wormlike in appearance, it is often called the vermiform appendix.

Some of the water (used in digestion) and electrolytes are reabsorbed by the caecum and the ascending colon. Although this is a relatively small amount of water reabsorption, it is crucial in maintaining proper fluid balance in the body.

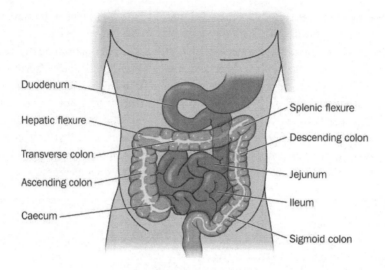

Figure 2.9 The intestines.

The colon can further be divided into four sections: ascending, transverse, descending and sigmoid. The *ascending* colon travels up the right side of the body to the level of the liver. The *transverse* colon travels across the abdomen just below the liver and the stomach. Bending downward near the spleen, the *descending* colon goes down the left side, where it becomes the sigmoid colon. The sigmoid (S-shaped) colon extends to the rectum. The rectum opens to the anal canal, which leads to the anus, which relaxes and opens to allow the passage of solid waste (faeces).

Peristalsis continues in the large intestine but at a slower rate. As these slower, intermittent waves move faecal matter toward the distal parts of the colon, water is removed, turning faeces from a watery soup to a semisolid mass. The material builds up in the sigmoid colon. The material is initially prevented from entering the rectum by the shape of the large bowel at this point – there is a sharp 'corner' between the colon and the rectum. Eventually a more powerful peristaltic wave occurs, and a significant quantity of material moves into the rectum.

The distension this causes to the rectal walls leads to the defecation reflex. This is a spinal reflex that causes the walls of the sigmoid colon and rectum to relax and those of the anal canal to open. At this point the individual becomes aware of the urge to defecate, and can choose whether to relax the external (voluntary) sphincter and defecate, or to tense it and avoid defecation.

Bacteria found in the large intestine helps to break down indigestible materials and produce B complex vitamins as well as most of the vitamin K that is required for blood clotting. Their presence also prevents other, potentially harmful, micro-organisms from colonising the large bowel.

Accessory organs

In addition to the salivary glands of the mouth, other accessory organs are necessary for digestion. These are the liver, gallbladder and pancreas.

Liver

The liver is located inferior to the diaphragm. The liver is the largest glandular organ in the body *and* the largest organ in the abdominopelvic cavity. The liver is divided into a larger right lobe and a smaller left lobe (Figure 2.10). The right lobe also has two smaller, inferior lobes. The liver receives about 1.5 litres of blood per minute from the hepatic portal vein (carrying blood full of the end products of digestion) and hepatic (referring to liver) artery (providing oxygen-rich blood).

The main functions of the liver include:

- Detoxification of harmful substances such as certain drugs and alcohol
- Creation of body heat
- Destruction of old blood cells, eliminating the pigment *bilirubin*. Bilirubin is eliminated in bile and gives faeces its distinctive colour
- Transamination of amino acids
- Formation of blood plasma proteins, for example *albumin* and *globulins*
- Production of the clotting factors *fibrinogen* and *prothrombin*.

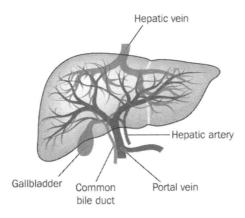

Figure 2.10 The liver.

■ Creation of the anticoagulant *heparin*
■ Manufacturing bile, needed for the digestion of fats
■ Storage and modification of fats for more efficient usage by the body's cells
■ Synthesis of *urea*, a by-product of protein metabolism
■ Storage of *glucose* as *glycogen*
■ Storage of iron and vitamins A, B$_{12}$, D, E and K
■ Production of cholesterol

Gallbladder

The gallbladder is a sac-shaped organ approximately 7.5-10 cm long located under the liver's right lobe (Figure 2.10). The role of the gallbladder is to store bile, but it also concentrates bile by reabsorbing water, making the bile six to ten times more concentrated than it was in the liver. When fatty foods enter the duodenum, the duodenum releases the hormone CCK (cholecystokinin). This release causes the smooth muscle walls of the gallbladder to contract and squeeze bile into the cystic duct, through the common bile duct and then into the duodenum.

Pancreas

The pancreas is located posterior to the stomach and extends laterally from the duodenum to the spleen (Figure 2.11). The exocrine portion of this organ secretes buffers and digestive enzymes through the *pancreatic duct* to the duodenum. These buffers are needed to neutralise the acidity of the chyme in the small intestine. With a pH ranging from 7.5 to 8.8, the chyme is neutralised, saving the intestinal wall from damage. This secretory action is activated by the release of hormones by the duodenum. The general digestive enzymes excreted by the pancreas are *carbohydrases* that work on sugars and starches, *lipases* that work on lipids (fats), *proteinases* that break down proteins, and *nucleases* that break down nucleic acids.

Activity
Review Chapters 5 and 10 and consider associated complications and implications for nursing care for patients that have pancreatitis.

Summary

The gastrointestinal system stretches from the mouth to the anus, and contains specialised structures and sections that are capable of digesting food, extracting useful material and excreting waste products. The gastrointestinal system is under

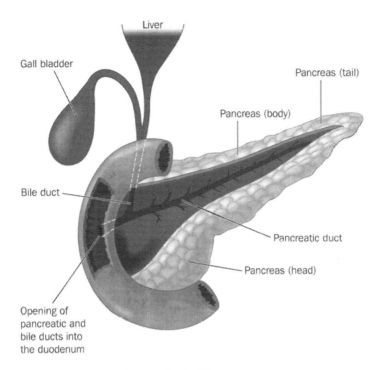

Figure 2.11 The pancreas.

hormonal control that is triggered once food enters the mouth. These hormones include gastrin, secretin and cholecystokinin, and are vital for the extraction of nutrients from the diet.

References

Apau, D. and Whiteing, N. (2011) Pre and post-operative nursing considerations of bariatric surgery. *Journal of Gastrointestinal Nursing*, **9**(3), 44–8.

Turner, M. and Ship, J. (2007) Dry mouth and its effects on the oral health of elderly people. *Journal of the American Dental Association*, **138**(1), 1S–20S.

Ship, J. A., Pillemer, S. R. and Baum, B. J. (2002) Xerostomia and the geriatric patient. *Journal of the American Geriatric Society*, **50**(3), 535–43.

Bibliography

Colbert, B., Ankley, J., Lee, K., Steggall, M. and Dingle, M. (2009) The gastrointestinal system. In: *Anatomy and Physiology for Nursing and Health Professionals* (eds. N. Colbert, J. Ankley, K. Lee, M. Steggall and M. Dingle). Pearson Education, Harlow.

Marieb, E. (2003) The digestive system and body metabolism. In: *Essentials of Human Anatomy and Physiology*, 7th edn (ed. E. Marieb), Chapter 14. Benjamin Cummings, London.

Marieb, E. and Hoehn, K. (2007) The digestive system. In: *Human Anatomy and Physiology*, 7th edn, Chapter 23. Pearson, Benjamin Cummings, London.

CHAPTER 3

Nutrition

Alison Coutts

Introduction

In this chapter the components of a healthy diet are considered, along with what each key nutrient provides for the body. Malnutrition (literally meaning 'bad nutrition') is discussed and the concept of protein-energy malnutrition is presented.

By reading this chapter and carrying out the proposed activities you should achieve the following learning outcomes:

- Improve your knowledge of what key nutrients are
- Understand the implications of reduced or excess nutrition
- Discuss the role of the nurse in promoting a healthy diet.

A healthy diet

A healthy diet is a balanced diet: one that provides all the required nutrients in approximately the required amounts each day. The diet would be safe, enjoyable and also fulfil social and cultural requirements.

So what nutrients are required? Nutrients can be classified as:

- Macro-nutrients: those that are required in significant quantities most days. These are proteins, lipids and carbohydrates.
- Micro-nutrients: those that are essential, but only required in tiny amounts. These are the vitamins and minerals.
- Water is not traditionally classified as a nutrient, but in view of its critical importance to health it is now often considered alongside nutrients.

Energy

Energy is required for all life functions. It is obviously required for the individual to exercise, but it is also needed for the heart to pump, the kidneys to filtrate and the lungs to ventilate. Energy is derived by cells from the macro-nutrients. These are taken up by the cell and processed through the tricarboxylic acid (TCA or Krebs) cycle to release adenosine triphosphate: the compound that the cell uses to do work.

$$C_6H_{12}O_6 + O_2 \rightarrow ATP + heat + H_2O + CO_2$$

Glucose + oxygen → adenosine triphosphate + heat + water + carbon dioxide

Energy is measured in joules (definitely not calories!). One joule is not a lot of energy, so it is usually stated in terms of kilojoules (kJ; one thousand joules) or even megajoules (MJ; one million joules).

Proteins

Proteins are made up of many – usually hundreds – of amino acids (Figure 3.1). The distinguishing characteristic of amino acids is that they all contain nitrogen.

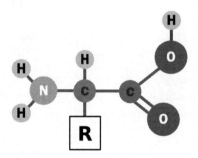

Figure 3.1 A generic amino acid (source: Wikipedia).

There are approximately 20 naturally occurring amino acids, although more can be artificially synthesised. Amino acids can further be classified as essential or non-essential. However, this term is misleading, as all are essential to health but some, the so called non-essential amino acids, can be synthesised from other amino acids. The 10 essential amino acids are histidine, isoleucine, leucine, lysine, methionine (or another sulphur-containing amino acid), casein, phenylalanine, threonine, tryptophan and valine. The non-essential amino acids are alanine, asparagine, aspartic acid, cysteine, glutamic acid, glutamine, glycine, proline, serine and tyrosine. There are two further complications: young people also require arginine (adults have the enzymes required for the synthesis of arginine) and tyrosine, which is produced from phenylalanine, so if the diet is deficient in the latter tyrosine will be required as well.

All these amino acids are essential for life: we need them for building most body tissues, but perhaps even more urgently we need them to manufacture chemicals essential for body functioning. Most enzymes, hormones and cell signalling compounds are primarily composed of amino acids. They are also present in cell membranes, where they act as receptors for these signalling compounds, and also provide channels regulating the movement of materials into and out of the cell.

Protein is widespread in the diet: meat, fish, dairy products, eggs, nuts, seeds, pulses and soya products all are good sources of protein. In the United Kingdom (UK) most people eat more protein than is absolutely necessary, which is about two portions of protein daily. Examples of a portion include:

- 100 g boneless meat (e.g. lean beef, lamb or pork)
- 100 g boneless poultry (e.g. chicken or turkey breast)
- 100 g fish (e.g. salmon, sardines or tuna)
- 2 medium eggs
- 3 tablespoons of seeds (e.g. sunflower or pumpkin seeds)
- 3 tablespoons of nuts (e.g. almonds or walnuts).

Activity

Think of your last meal (or the next one). What proportion of your meal contained protein? Did you weigh it or estimate it? Consider what the risks of estimating protein intake might be.

If intake of protein is marginal, it may be necessary to ensure that the patient is receiving the required amounts of all the essential amino acids. There are a number of ways of assessing the quality of proteins. A high-quality protein would contain all the amino acids in the appropriate amounts and in an easily digestible form. Biological value (BV) is the concept used to assess how much of a protein food can be used by the body. If the BV is 100% that would be perfect as all the protein could be used because the profile of amino acids exactly matches that required. Whole egg has a BV of 93.7% and is the best single food; milk has a BV of 84.5%. Proteins from animal sources tend to best match those required by humans, who are, after all, animals. However meat, particularly red meat, is also high in saturated fats, and many people prefer to take more plant proteins. These are more likely to be deficient in one or more essential amino acids, referred to as the limiting amino acid. Therefore people who get most or all of their protein from plant sources need to eat a wider variety of foods. It is interesting to note that many traditional dishes appear to offer complementary food sources, presumably without our ancestors knowing the science for this; thus wheat is deficient in lysine but rich in methionine. Beans, on the other hand do not have much methionine but are rich in lysine, so eating beans on toast makes for a nutritious meal! Similarly macaroni and cheese offers a meal of high biological value.

Proteins can be used by the cells for energy. Each gram of pure protein yields 17 kJ of energy. It is sometimes fashionable to take a very high protein diet but one that is low in other nutrients. In this instance the individual is forced to use protein for energy. However, there is little evidence for the suggested health benefits of this type of diet and such a diet is expensive!

Lipids

Lipids are often referred to as 'fat', but fats are solids at room temperature, whereas oils, which are also lipids, are liquid at room temperature. Most of the lipids we eat, and almost all those in our bodies, are triglycerides (Figure 3.2).

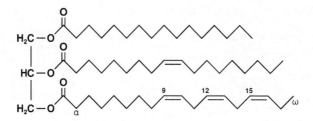

Figure 3.2 A triglyceride (source: Wikipedia).

These are composed of a glycerol 'backbone' with three fatty acids attached. It is the nature of the fatty acids that makes one lipid different from another.

Fatty acids are essential for life. There are hundreds of different types of fatty acid. Of these, two – alpha-linolenic acid and linoleic acid – are essential in the diet. Three other fatty acids are defined as being conditionally essential, that is they are required in certain situations; these are gamma linolenic acid, lauric acid and palmitoleic acid. The majority of fatty acids found in foods are composed of a single, un-branched, chain of many (often very many) carbon atoms with hydrogen atoms attached. They can be classified as saturated or unsaturated: carbon is able to attach easily to four other atoms. In a fatty acid the carbons (except those on either end of the chain) will be attached to a carbon on either side, then up to two hydrogen atoms. A saturated fatty acid is where all the 'spaces' are taken up with an atom of hydrogen. An unsaturated fatty acid is one where there are some 'vacancies'; in this case the carbons will form a double bond with each other. A mono unsaturated fatty acid has just one double bond, whilst a polyunsaturated fatty acid has several double bonds.

Fatty acids have multiple functions in health, and are involved in regulating immune function, facilitating neurological function and homeostasis. They are also a very rich source of energy, yielding 37 kJ per gram, that is more than twice any other nutrient (except alcohol, which is not legally defined as a nutrient). It is this that has given them a reputation for being 'fattening'. They are also associated with the development of atheroma and the attendant cardiovascular diseases. However, this is not strictly true, as some lipids are actually protective from cardiovascular disease. These are the mono-unsaturated fatty acids, i.e. where there is just one double bond in the molecule. A diet high in monounsaturated fatty acids leads to the formation of high-density lipo-proteins, which may actually reverse atheroma and other damage to the circulating system. This group of fatty acids can be further sub-classified according to the position of that double bond, the most important are in the third position (omega-3) or sixth position (omega-6). Omega-6 fatty acids tend to be abundant in our diet as they are present in cooking oil, whereas omega-3 fatty acids (including alpha linolenic acid) are less abundant, but they are present in oily fish. The body will absorb and metabolise omega-3 and omega-6 fatty acids in proportion to that in the diet, so having much more omega six fatty acids present may lead to a relative deficiency of omega-3 fatty acids. Many people choose to take supplements of omega-3 fatty acids, believing that they have widespread health benefits. Although there is a lack of evidence for some of these claims, they do appear to be of benefit in controlling allergic conditions (Calder, 2006). However, it should be noted that all lipids have equally high energy yields.

Carbohydrates

Carbohydrates are composed of carbon, hydrogen and oxygen. Unlike the other macro-nutrients, their only function is to provide energy, although some of the components are used in a regulatory function. They are classified according to how many 'sugar units' are in the molecule: thus monosaccharides, such as glucose or fructose, are made up of just one sugar unit; disaccharides, such as sucrose (table sugar), are made up of two; and polysaccharides are made up of several sugar units. Monosaccharides and disaccharides are small, simple molecules that taste sweet and are easily broken down to yield glucose which the cells can readily convert into ATP. Complex carbohydrates, on the other hand, are large and chemically complex molecules with multiple chemical bonds, which taste bland and take a lot of time to break down. This concept is summarised by the foods 'glycaemic index'. Simple sugars provide a 'quick energy boost', but can be associated with wide alterations in blood sugar. Complex carbohydrates, on the other hand, usually have a low glycaemic index: they are slow to yield energy, but provide a steadier and more sustained support to blood glucose levels.

Carbohydrates are abundant in the diet. They include most sweet-tasting foods and also bulky but bland foods like potatoes, pasta, bread and rice. They yield 17 kJ of energy per gram, the same as proteins. We are now encouraged to obtain 60–80% of our energy from carbohydrates and only 20–40% from lipids, but most people take much more lipid than this.

Minerals

Minerals occur in the natural world around us – the soil and rocks. Animals will often lick rocks to obtain their minerals, but humans prefer to take them in either with water that has run over these rocks, or by eating material (plants and animals) that has incorporated this water! Many minerals are recognised as essential for health; they often have very specific roles, involved in just a handful of biochemical pathways.

One critical mineral is iron. Adult men required about 7 mg of iron daily, but women of childbearing years require about 15 mg, due to the additional requirements of menstruation. About 1 in 20 men and older women experience iron deficiency anaemia, but the figure for women of childbearing age is between one in four and two in five (Scientific Advisory Committee on Nutrition, 2009). This makes it the most common nutritional deficiency in the UK, with women, pre-school children and older adults at particular risk. The consequences can be serious, with anaemia the most obvious effect, leading to tiredness and intolerance of exercise, but also to learning difficulties in children and delayed motor development. The richest source is red meat, but this is also rich in saturated fats, and other sources should be considered, such as dried fruit, leafy green vegetables, nuts and seeds.

Other minerals include calcium, needed for neurological function and to maintain bone density, sodium, potassium and phosphorous. This list may not be exhaustive, as zinc is widely recognised as having a role in supporting the immune system. However, a Cochrane Review (Singh and Das, 2011) found that the benefits of supplementation were so small as to not warrant the expense and side-effects. This is typical of popular claims for many minerals, our knowledge of minerals in health in increasing all the time, but nurses need to interpret some claims with caution, as many lack good quality evidence.

Vitamins

Vitamins, like minerals, are essential but are required in only small amounts. Vitamins are usually large, complex molecules and, unlike minerals, are synthesised by plants and animals, but humans lack the enzymes necessary to synthesise them, so need to take them in the diet.

Vitamins are often classified as being water-soluble (vitamin C and the B complex of vitamins) or lipid soluble (vitamins A, D, E and K).

Of these, vitamin C (ascorbic acid) is the vitamin that is required in largest amounts. We need between 70 and 100 mg daily. It is abundant in fresh fruit and vegetables, particularly those with a strong colour. Severe lack of vitamin C leads to scurvy, a most unpleasant and ultimately fatal disease characterised by a breakdown of collagen. However, in modern Britain most people take in adequate vitamin C. There are several claims that vitamin C can cure all sorts of diseases, particularly infections and those involved in the immune response, but the evidence for this is, once again, sketchy: there is no evidence for instance, that very high doses of vitamin C will prevent the common cold, but it may shorten its duration (Hamilla *et al.*, 2010).

Activity
What makes up a healthy diet? Think about the advice you might give a patient/client and the factors that might influence your advice (e.g. access to food type, cost, food preparation).

Definition of malnutrition

Most people understand malnutrition to mean deficiency. People may think of television news items of people starving in refugee camps as suffering from malnutrition. However, malnutrition means bad nutrition, so any form of poor nutritional intake could be defined as malnutrition. Thus an obese person may also be suffering from malnutrition. Refer to Figure 3.3 for examples of under- and over-nutrition associated with malnutrition.

The nurse is advised to refer to under- or over-nutrition, rather than malnutrition, so that she/he is always understood. A further important distinction needs to be made, particularly as regards under nutrition, and that is whether the person is suffering from a lack of macro-nutrients or micro-nutrients. Under-nutrition of the macro-nutrients is the classic image that many people have of malnutrition. This is often referred to as protein-energy malnutrition. Such people

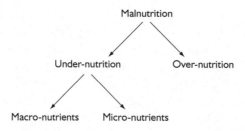

Figure 3.3 Protein-energy malnutrition

are also often severely deficient in vitamins and minerals, but this is dwarfed by the life-threatening shortage of lipid, protein and energy. This type of malnutrition is usually only seen in the UK as secondary to other disorders, such as malabsorption syndromes. In contrast, under-nutrition of some of the micro-nutrients, particularly iron, is very common and leads to many sub-clinical health problems.

In contrast, over-nutrition is a very urgent problem in the UK. It is often thought to be a problem associated with affluence, but the reality is more complex than this (Dahley *et al.*, 2010). Obesity is associated with many negative impacts on health. Presently an effective public health strategy is being actively sought to address obesity in the UK.

Activity
Identify the prevalence of malnutrition in your local area. Which is more common, under- or over-nutrition? Why might this be the case?

Dehydration

Whilst plenty of people survive with under-nutrition, a lack of water is a very dangerous situation. The recommended intake of water in the UK is approximately 1.2 litres a day, and more if it is very hot or if the individual is working very hard. In such circumstances up to 500 ml every half hour may be required (NHS Choices, 2010). In addition, most people will obtain water from the normal metabolism of food.

Water loss is a dangerous effect of diarrhoea; particularly in the very young. In the UK people are fortunate in that good quality drinking water is almost always available from the tap; there is no need to buy expensive 'mineral waters', except, possibly, for their taste. Caffeinated drinks are mild diuretics, so if these are taken in large amounts then the person needs to drink a little more than 1.2 litres of water each day.

It is currently fashionable to drink significantly more than the recommended volume of water, which is usually unnecessary and could cause health problems. Water intoxication can occur if extreme amounts of water are taken, particularly in the absence of sodium intake. Water intoxication causes the brain to swell and ultimately can lead to death.

Screening and assessment of nutritional status

It is now widely accepted that many hospital patients are undernourished on admission to hospital, and that this actually gets worse during their stay (Hafsteinsdottir *et al.*, 2010). This has implications for their prognosis as, at the very least, it will prolong their hospital stay (Caccialanza *et al.*, 2010). Most hospitals therefore routinely carry out some form of screening for malnutrition on admission to health care and, ideally, regularly afterwards. However, obtaining a meaningful dietary assessment can be difficult.

Dietary assessment

Dietary assessment involves the nurse asking the patient about their diet and then making a judgement as to whether it is adequate. This approach is fraught with difficulty. It is difficult to remember what was taken (can you remember what you had for lunch two days ago?) and even more difficult to assess the nutritional load of the food taken. It may be possible to use this means of assessing a diet for one or two nutrients, or for identifying grossly deficient diets, but is of limited value in most cases.

Biometric measurements

Biometric measurements involve taking measurements from the individual. This is usually measurement of height and weight, but it can also include skin fold thickness and/or arm circumference. This approach has, in the past, been used very successfully to identify malnourished children and can be of value in assessing adults.

Physiological and biochemical measurements

Physiological measurements can reflect a person's nutritional status. Subsequently, immune function may reflect how well nourished people are. However, there are not many validated trials to substantiate how reliable these measurements are.

Biochemical measurements can be taken for individual nutrients. Thus haemoglobin levels can reflect a person's recent iron intake, and the Schilling test can show whether someone is deficient in vitamin B_{12}. This works well in these cases, but it is not possible to screen everybody for every nutrient. There is a limit to the number of tests that can be performed. In addition, there are methodological problems, as at present there is not enough research data to substantiate what is 'normal'.

Malnutrition Universal Screening Tool (MUST)

The Malnutrition Universal Screening Tool (MUST) is a validated tool developed in the UK by several health professionals working together (Malnutrition Advisory Group, 2011). It takes a variety of approaches to assess nutritional status, including weight and height, recent (unplanned) weight loss and clinical illness. From this information the nurse derives a score to indicate whether the patient is at risk of malnutrition or of developing malnutrition. It should be stressed that MUST is a screening tool, not a full assessment tool. It is used to assess individuals quickly and easily, perhaps upon admission to healthcare; those people who are identified as being at risk will require further assessment. Although MUST does provide some ideas as to how to proceed with the care of these people, it can only offer an initial screening and not a full diagnostic assessment.

Activity
Review the MUST tool (http://www.bapen.org.uk/pdfs/must/must_full. pdf) and explanatory booklet (http://www.bapen.org.uk/pdfs/must/must_ explan.pdf). Are these used in your clinical area? How would you introduce them into practice?

Food poisoning

Strictly speaking, the intake of anything that causes harm could be classified as food poisoning. However, the term has come to mean eating food colonised by bacteria that cause illness. Food poisoning can cause a great deal of harm. There are over 9 million cases of gastro-enteritis in the UK each year, and this is steadily increasing. People affected by food poisoning experience nausea, vomiting, diarrhoea and abdominal cramps. The timing of the onset of these symptoms is a characteristic of the causative organism, but is usually within a few hours to two days after the intake of the food. Most people experience a spontaneous recovery, but food poisoning causes 100-200 deaths per annum in the UK. Very young, very old and immune-suppressed individuals are at particular risk. Most deaths are the result of dehydration, so nurses must be vigilant for signs of this, particularly when vulnerable people become unwell. In cases of dehydration, very young, older and immune-suppressed individuals may require intravenous fluids.

Causative organisms

There are a variety of organisms commonly associated with food poisoning. The most common organism associated with food poisoning is *Campylobacter*. This is a relatively new cause, and fortunately rarely causes dangerous illness. The most likely source is undercooked chicken, but it can also come from other meats and unpasteurised milk. It rarely causes big outbreaks, as it does not replicate at room temperature. It can be passed between people if hand hygiene is poor (Good Food UK, 2009).

There are many strains of *Salmonella* that can cause food poisoning. Many uncooked chickens are contaminated with *Salmonella*. It can survive freezing, but fortunately not high temperatures. *Salmonella* originated in cattle, but now is found in many farm animals and may be associated with cramped, stressful conditions.

Many strains of *Escherichia coli* live harmlessly in the large bowel of most people. However, if it gets into food, usually through poor hygiene, it can cause severe illness. Fortunately, severe illness is rare. There was a notorious incident in Scotland where several hundred elderly people became ill after eating beef contaminated with one strain of *E. coli*, called *E. coli* 0157 (British Medical Journal News, 1996).

Activity

List the most common causes of food poisoning. Why are some pathogens more prone to cause food poisoning than others?

Prevention

Most cases are caused by poor food hygiene and are therefore preventable. Approximately 17% of cases of food poisoning originate in the home (Good Food UK, 2009). Forty-four per cent originate in meals bought in restaurants and as 'take aways', and the remainder are cases where contamination has occurred somewhere in the food chain. Rules relating to the handling of food to avoid food poisoning are logical and include:

- Always wash hands thoroughly before preparing food, after going to the toilet and after handling pets
- Keep kitchen work surfaces clean
- Ensure that food is defrosted completely before cooking (unless product is intended to be cooked from frozen)
- Keep pets away from food
- Ensure that food is cooked thoroughly before eating. Meat shouldn't have any pink bits
- Serve reheated food piping hot
- Keep raw meat and fish covered and store at the bottom of the refrigerator
- Store cooked and raw food separate, and do not use the same utensils on them
- Store all perishable foods below 5 °C
- Keep raw food covered
- Rinse fruit and vegetables under running water before eating
- Throw away any food that is past its 'use by' date, doesn't smell right and/or has fungus on it.

Food poverty, food security and the politics of food

It seems a travesty that while in modern Britain people have access to more and better food than ever before there are widespread concerns about the quality of people's diets. For this reason, a public health strategy is urgently being sought by the UK government.

It is known that the quality of a child's diet is profoundly influenced by their mother's attitude to food; even after confounding factors (such as affluence). This influence persists well into adulthood (Fisk *et al.*, 2011) and subsequently influences the foods that they will provide for their own children. Lang *et al.* (2009) explored why it is that, in a county of increasing wealth and in the face of advances in scientific and medical understanding, people are apparently still suffering from food inequality. It is viewed that the nation's health is being systematically damaged by problems such as obesity (Dahley *et al.*, 2010).

Lang *et al.* (2009) researched the concept of food deserts. The concept of a food desert is an area where there is a shortage of shops selling food that is both good in quality and at a fair price. They found that where there are food deserts there are often plenty of fast food outlets, whose food is frequently characterised by high salt and fat content and which is low in micro-nutrients. Food deserts are often found where the resident population is on low incomes. The poor quality of food compounds the low-income population's already damaged life chances. People on lower incomes traditionally spend a higher portion of their incomes on food and they are particularly vulnerable to fluctuations in the availability of food and the price they have to pay for it. Taking all of the aforementioned into consideration means that malnourishment is a significant concern in this population. Lang *et al.* (2009) argued that food, and its cost and quality, cannot be left to chance or to market forces. It is the responsibility of the food industry and those who produce, prepare and market food, as well as the government, to actively address these inequalities. Clearly, in such circumstances the nurse has a significant role to play in monitoring people's nutritional status and educating people about healthy eating habits.

Summary

This chapter has considered the elements that make up nutrients and what each nutrient provides the human body. Nutrition and malnutrition have been discussed and the differences between over- and under-nutrition outlined. Food poisoning, which is very common, has been outlined and the common causative pathogens discussed. In addition, food poverty, food security and the politics of food have been reflected upon. It has been identified that the nurse has a significant role to play in monitoring the nutritional status of people and educating people about healthy eating habits.

References

Calder, P. C. (2006) n–3 polyunsaturated fatty acids, inflammation, and inflammatory diseases. *American Journal of Clinical Nutrition*, **83**(6), S1505–19.

British Medical Journal News (1996) *E. coli* kills five people in Scotland. *British Medical Journal*, **313**(7070), 1424.

Caccialanza, R., Klerzy, C., Cereda, E., Cameletti, B., Bonoldi, A., Barnadi, C., Marinelli, M. and Dionigi, P. (2010) Nutritional parameters associated with prolonged hospital stay among adult ambulatory patients. *Canadian Medical Association Journal*, **182**(17), 1843–9.

Dahley, D., Gordon-Larkson, P., Popkin, B., Kaufman, J. S. and Adair, L. S. (2010) Associations between multiple indicators of socioeconomic status and obesity in young Filipinos vary by gender, urbanicity and indicators used. *Journal of Nutrition*, **140**(2), 366–70.

Fisk, C. M., Crozier, S. R., Inskip, H. M., Godfrey, K. M., Cooper, C. and Robinson, S. M. (2011) Influence on the quality of young children's diets: the importance of maternal food choices. *British Journal of Nutrition*, **105**(2), 287–96.

Good Food UK (2009) *Food poisoning*. http://www.basicfoodhygiene.co.uk/food_poisoning.htm (accessed 15 March 2011)

Hafsteinsdottir, T., Mosselman, M. and Schoneveld, C. (2010) Malnutrition in hospitalised neurological patients approximately doubles in ten days of hospitalisation. *Journal of Clinical Nursing*, **19**(5–6), 639–48.

Hamilla, H., Chalker, E. and Douglas, B. (Cochrane Acute Respiratory Infections Group) (2010) *Vitamin C for Preventing and Alleviating the Common Cold.* http://summaries.cochrane.org/CD000980/vitamin-c-for-preventing-and-treating-the-common-cold (accessed 24 November 2011).

Lang, T., Barling, D. and Caraher, M. (eds.) (2009) *Food Policy: Integrating Health, Environment and Society.* Oxford University Press, Oxford.

Malnutrition Advisory Group (2011) *Malnutrition Universal Screening Tool.* http://www.bapen.org.uk/pdfs/must/must_full.pdf. (accessed 15 March 2011).

NHS Choices (2010) *Dehydration.* http://www.nhs.uk/conditions/dehydration/pages/introduction.aspx (accessed 15 March 2011).

Scientific Advisory Committee on Nutrition (2009) *Draft Report on Nutrition and Health.* Food Standards Agency, UK.

Singh, M. and Das, R. R. (Cochrane Acute Respiratory Infections Group) (2011) *Zinc for the Common Cold.* http://summaries.cochrane.org/CD001364/zinc-for-the-common-cold (accessed 24 November 2011).

CHAPTER 4

Upper gastrointestinal complaints

Warren Chapman

Introduction

This chapter considers complaints of the upper gastrointestinal (GI) tract. Conditions of the oesophagus, stomach and duodenum will be discussed. Conditions of the lower GI tract will be discussed in Chapter 5. By reading this chapter and carrying out the proposed activities you should achieve the following learning outcomes:

- Improve your knowledge of the various upper GI complaints
- Have a better understanding of the management options available
- Understand the diagnostic tests patients with upper GI symptoms may undergo
- Be able to discuss the lifestyle changes some patients with upper GI complaints may find beneficial.

Presenting signs and symptoms

Patients with upper GI complaints can present with the following signs and symptoms: dyspepsia, nausea and vomiting, dysphagia, odynophagia, weight loss, haematemesis, melaena, waterbrash, anaemia and anorexia.

Definitions

- *Dyspepsia* means poor digestion. The term describes a group of symptoms including epigastric pain, heartburn, nausea or vomiting, early satiety (feeling full quickly during a meal) and bloating. Dyspepsia-type symptoms can be functional in nature (i.e. they do not represent any organic disease), or they can indicate a wide variety of problems, including peptic (gastric, duodenal or oesophageal) ulceration, cancer and gall bladder disease, as well as heart or musculo-skeletal problems.

■ *Nausea and vomiting* is a complex syndrome. Vomiting is also called emesing (*emesis* means vomit). Nausea will often precede vomiting. The vomiting reflex is controlled by the medulla oblongata in the brain. It involves the stimulation of respiratory, skeletal and gastrointestinal muscles to forcibly eject gastric and even duodenal contents out of the mouth. It is the body's means of protecting itself from ingested toxic substances. However, it may occur as a result of peptic ulcer disease and could indicate gastric outflow obstruction. Vomiting can also be anxiety related. This is known as psychogenic vomiting.

■ *Dysphagia* is when foods gets stuck on swallowing and can indicate gastro-oesophageal reflux (reflux of, usually acidic, gastric contents into the oesophagus), cancer or other problems related to the neck and thoracic cavity.

■ *Odynophagia* means pain on swallowing. It may be caused by infection with *Candida* (thrush), herpes or cytomegalovirus. Such infections could indicate the presence of HIV. Sudden onset of odynophagia could also indicate impaction of a foreign body (e.g. a fishbone).

■ *Weight loss* may indicate cancer or gastric/duodenal ulceration. It is important to note whether patients have been dieting (i.e. intentional weight loss) and also to calculate how much weight has been lost over what period of time.

■ *Haematemesis* means vomiting of blood and may be caused by peptic ulceration, cancer or prolonged vomiting. It may be bright red or look like coffee grounds due to the blood being altered (partially digested).

■ *Melaena* is the passage of stools containing altered blood. Often it is black, tarry and foul smelling. This can indicate peptic ulceration or cancer.

■ *Waterbrash* is the regurgitation of sour or tasteless fluid into the mouth and can indicate ulcers or gastro-oesophageal reflux disease.

■ *Anaemia* is a drop to below normal of haemoglobin in the blood. The normal range for a man is 13.5–17.5 g/dl and for a woman is 11.5–15.5 g/dl. Anaemia could indicate blood loss as a result of ulceration, vascular (blood vessel) lesions, cancer or polyps (abnormal growths of tissue projecting from the mucous membranes). Other causes of anaemia can include menstrual blood loss, reduced intake (e.g. of iron, folate, vitamin B_{12} (may occur with vegetarians or vegans)), malabsorption (e.g. coeliac disease), Crohn's disease or pernicious anaemia.

■ *Anorexia* means poor appetite and may be associated with weight loss.

Activity

Ask if you can spend time observing a gastroenterology clinic. This may be conducted by a gastroenterology medical consultant or a specialist nurse.

Think about the various signs and symptoms the patients present with and note the investigations and management plans that the specialist agrees with the patients.

Consider the impact that these symptoms have on each patient's life. Think about ways in which each patient may be able to make their lifestyle healthier.

Epidemiology

The percentage of people with dyspepsia in the Western world is estimated to be 23–41% (British Society of Gastroenterology (BSG), 2002) and makes up 40% of all gastroenterological consultations (Moayyedi *et al.*, 2009). It has been estimated that at least £100 million per year is spent from the NHS budget on drugs to treat the symptoms. Worldwide the figure equates to £2 billion (Forgacs and Loganayagam, 2008). The problem is that upper GI symptoms can indicate anything from functional dyspepsia to cancer. Cancer of the oesophagus is the fifth largest cause of cancer death in the UK and is increasing in incidence annually (Cancer Research UK, 2009). Cancer of the stomach is the eighth largest cancer killer in males and the thirteenth in females. It has more than halved in incidence since the mid 1970s (Cancer Research UK, 2007). The challenge is to ensure that dyspepsia symptoms are assessed adequately, ensuring that cancers are diagnosed, whilst at the same time ensuring that the medical system is not overwhelmed by investigating every single case of dyspepsia. Consequently, in the UK, the National Institute for Health and Clinical Excellence (NICE) has produced guidance on the management of adults suffering with dyspepsia (NICE, 2004) (see Box 4.1). The guidance advocates treating dyspepsia symptoms first with either proton pump inhibitor (PPI) tablets (see Table 4.1) or *Helicobacter pylori* (a bacteria that can cause dyspepsia and ulceration in the stomach and duodenum) eradication treatment, unless the patient presents with symptoms indicative of cancer (i.e. weight loss, iron deficiency anaemia, epigastric mass or persistent vomiting).

Box 4.1 National Institute for Health and Clinical Excellence (NICE) Dyspepsia Guidelines 2004 (updated 2005)

Referral for endoscopy

Review medications for possible causes of dyspepsia (for example, calcium antagonists, nitrates, theophyllines, biphosphates, corticosteroids and non-steroidal anti-inflammatory drugs (NSAIDs). In patients requiring referral suspend NSAID use.

Urgent specialist referral for endoscopic investigation (within 2 weeks) is indicated for patients of any age with dyspepsia when presenting with any of the following: chronic gastrointestinal bleeding, progressive unintentional weight loss, progressive difficulty swallowing, persistent vomiting, iron deficiency anaemia, epigastric mass or suspicious barium meal.

Routine endoscopic investigation of patients of any age, presenting with dyspepsia and without alarm signs, is not necessary. However, in patients aged 55 years and older with unexplained and persistent recent onset of dyspepsia alone, an urgent referral for endoscopy should be made.

Interventions for un-investigated dyspepsia

Initial therapeutic strategies for dyspepsia are empirical treatment with a proton pump inhibitor (PPI) or testing for and treating *H. pylori*. There is currently insufficient evidence to guide which should be offered first. A 2 week washout period following PPI use is necessary before testing for *H. pylori* with a breath test or stool antigen test.

Interventions for gastro-oesophageal reflux disease (GORD)

Offer patients who have GORD a full dose PPI for 1 or 2 months.

If symptoms recur following initial treatment offer a PPI at the lowest possible dose to control symptoms, with a limited number of repeat prescriptions.

Interventions for peptic ulcer disease

Offer *H. pylori* eradication therapy to *H. pylori*-positive patients who have peptic ulcer disease.

For patients using NSAIDS with diagnosed peptic ulcer, stop the use of NSAIDS where possible. Offer full dose PPI or H2RA therapy for 2 months to these patients and if *H. pylori* are present, subsequently offer eradication therapy.

Interventions for non-ulcer dyspepsia

Management of endoscopically determined non-ulcer dyspepsia involves initial treatment for *H. pylori* if present followed by symptomatic management and periodic monitoring. Re-testing after eradication should not be offered routinely, although the information it provides may be valued by individual patients.

Reviewing patient care

Offer patients requiring long-term management of symptoms of dyspepsia an annual review of their condition. Encourage them to try stepping down or stopping treatment.

A return to self-treatment with antacid and/or alginate therapy (either prescribed or purchased over-the-counter and taken as required) may be appropriate.

H. pylori testing and eradication

H. pylori can be initially detected using either a carbon-13 urea breath test or a stool antigen test, or laboratory-based serology where its performance has been locally validated.

Office based serological tests for *H. pylori* cannot be recommended because of their inadequate performance.

For patients who test positive, provide a 7 day, twice daily course of treatment consisting of a full dose PPI with either metronidazole 400 mg and clarithromycin 250 mg or amoxicillin 1 g and clarithromycin 500 mg.

Activity

Talk with your friends and relations and see how many of them have suffered with symptoms of dyspepsia. Ask what the symptoms are, what makes them worse and what gives relief. Consider how the NICE guidance relates to them. You may need to offer them advice to visit their General Practitioner.

Investigations

Upper GI endoscopy

Nowadays this is a very common method of investigating upper GI symptoms. It is sometimes called a gastroscopy or an OGD, which stands for oesophagogastroduodenoscopy. The test involves passing a flexible tube containing a video camera, through the mouth, down the oesophagus through the stomach and into the duodenum. The endoscopist then carefully moves the endoscope examining all surfaces. Biopsies and images can be taken. Additionally therapy can be initiated during the test, such as injection or heat therapy to stop an ulcer from bleeding, or a dilatation to stretch a stricture (narrowing) in the oesophagus. Patients can have a sedative injection for the test, though nowadays it is very common for patients to have the test with just a spray of local anaesthetic to the oropharynx (back of the throat). This test is usually carried out as a day case, though patients may have it performed as an emergency, for instance if they present with haematemesis or melaena. Patients should have nothing to eat or drink for at least six hours prior to the test. This ensures the stomach is empty and allows good views. Additionally it also prevents aspiration of stomach contents into the lungs. Patients should be assessed before endoscopy to ensure they are fit for the procedure. Patients with respiratory or heart problems may be at risk, particularly if they are having the test with a sedative which can impair respiratory and cardiac function (Royal College of Anaesthetists, 2001). Risks of endoscopy can also include perforation of the upper GI tract or significant bleeding (British Society of Gastroenterology, 2006). Refer to Chapter 9 for additional information on imaging.

Activity
- Ask if you can spend a half day on the endoscopy unit observing an upper GI endoscopy list. Patients will be asked to give permission for you to observe.
- Note the reasons why each patient has been referred (indication).
- List the various diagnoses made during the endoscopy list.
- Make a note of how the patient tolerated the procedure and whether they had the test with a sedative injection or local anaesthetic spray. If you were to undergo the procedure, which option would you choose?
- Reflect on the various concerns the patient had on attending for this procedure.

Radiological tests
Tests used in investigating upper GI complaints include ultrasound, CT scan, barium meal/swallow and magnetic resonance imaging (MRI). These are dealt with in detail in Chapter 9.

Blood tests

Blood tests can indicate upper GI complaints. A full blood count (FBC) can show if the patient has anaemia which can indicate ulceration or cancer; although anaemia may indicate a cancer of the lower GI tract as well. A serology test can also be taken to see if the body has produced antibodies to *H. pylori*. Additionally abnormalities in liver function tests (LFTs) can show problems with the biliary system which may cause symptoms of upper GI complaints.

Oesophageal manometry

Oesophageal manometry involves passing a special catheter through the nose and into the oesophagus. It is a means of testing the different pressures along the length of the oesophagus. It can show whether the oesophageal muscles are working correctly, either to allow adequate swallowing or to stop excessive reflux of stomach contents into the oesophagus.

Oesophageal pH monitoring

This is often carried out at the same time as manometry. A catheter placed, via the nose, into the oesophagus measures the acidity within the oesophagus. The catheter usually stays in place for 24 hours and is connected to a special recording device which the patient carries around with them. A recording of the acidity within the oesophagus over a prolonged period is then obtained. It can be used to assess the level of acid reflux from the stomach and is useful when surgery for gastro-oesophageal reflux is being considered.

Diagnoses

Gastro-oesophageal reflux

This is the reflux of the acidic contents of the stomach into the oesophagus. Symptoms are commonly retrosternal (behind the breastbone) pain or discomfort. This can sometimes radiate through to the back between the shoulder blades. It can occasionally be difficult to distinguish between pain caused by gastro-oesophageal reflux disease or cardiac pain, though cardiac pain may be distinguishable by being worse on exertion, while discomfort from reflux can be positional (i.e. when lying flat or bending forward). Symptoms may be worse at night when the patient is lying flat, as acid will more easily reflux into the oesophagus in this position. Symptoms may also include a cough or asthma which is worse at night as a result of acid refluxing up the oesophagus and into the upper respiratory tract. Reflux symptoms may also be worse after large meals. Fatty foods are also thought to induce reflux. Foods such as chocolate and peppers may make it worse too. Additionally, obesity

49

can impact on reflux symptoms, as excess fat around the abdomen can increase pressure on the stomach and cause acid to reflux into the oesophagus.

When patients with gastro-oesophageal reflux undergo endoscopy, various degrees of oesophagitis or ulceration may be seen. Very severe oesophagitis or ulceration can result in the oesophagus bleeding into the stomach. This may result in haematemesis. Severe oesophagitis can lead to scarring of the oesophagus and strictures. Patients with strictures often complain of dysphagia. Some strictures may be stretched during endoscopy. Solitary oesophageal ulcers should be biopsied on endoscopy, as they can be cancerous.

Gastro-oesophageal reflux can be treated in the following ways:

- *Lifestyle measures.* Cutting down on fatty foods. Keeping a food diary to see which foods exacerbate the condition. Losing weight. Using more pillows at bedtime or raising the head of the bed.
- *Drug treatments.* These include PPIs, H2RA receptors, raft alginates and antacids and motility stimulants (see Table 4.1)
- *Surgical treatment.* A common surgical procedure is Nissan's fundoplication, which involves wrapping the top of the stomach around the bottom of the oesophagus to tighten the junction and reduce the amounts of acid refluxing upwards. This can often be done as a day case with laparoscopic (keyhole surgery). However, the success rate is variable so it is often performed as a last resort when other means of controlling reflux have failed.

Barrett's oesophagus

Barrett's oesophagus is also called Columnar Lined Oesophagus or CLO. It occurs when part of the usual squamous cell lining of the oesophagus is replaced with columnar cells (usually found in the stomach). This is believed to be a response to acid reflux. Current estimates suggest that 0.5–1% of patients with Barrett's oesophagus per year will develop oesophageal adenocarcinoma, which is a form of oesophageal cancer (Ackroyd *et al.*, 1997; Caygill *et al.*, 2004; Fitzgerald, 2005). The cellular changes typical of Barrett's oesophagus can be seen in the oesophagus on endoscopy. However, to test the diagnosis, biopsies must be taken. If these prove Barrett's oesophagus, then patients who are fit enough should be offered surveillance, where they return for endoscopy and biopsy every two years (British Society of Gastroenterology, 2005). That way any cancerous type changes may be detected earlier and subsequently treatment or surgery can be undertaken. Patients with Barrett's oesophagus should take PPI tablets to help reduce acid reflux and the progression of the disease. They should also be encouraged to implement the lifestyle advice for gastro-oesophageal reflux.

Activity

Visit the website of Core (http://www.corecharity.org.uk/), a charity which works with the British Society of Gastroenterology to fund research and provide patient information. Look in the patient information section and see how many leaflets you can find relating to upper GI complaints. These will be a useful resource for your patients; additionally they will also be an excellent learning aid for yourself.

Achalasia

Achalasia is characterised by dysphagia or regurgitation of undigested food. It may sometimes be accompanied by chest pain. Drug treatments are available for it, though often oesophageal dilatation is used. In some cases an operation on the muscles of the oesophagus, called a myotomy may be performed.

Oesophageal pouches, diverticulii and webs

These are anatomical variations which may sometimes be found in the oesophagus. Diverticulii are outpouchings of the mucosa caused by weaknesses in the muscle wall. Some of these pouches can be quite large. Symptoms of these may include dysphagia and regurgitation of undigested food. Barium swallow can be used to make a diagnosis. Surgical treatment may be necessary.

Webs are thin membranes of mucosa that can cause a narrowing. Many patients may not know they have a web, though dysphagia may be experienced occasionally (e.g. with tough meat). Webs may be seen on endoscopy or barium swallow. A dilatation of the oesophagus can be performed for persistent symptoms.

Mallory–Weiss tear

This is a tear of the mucosa at the bottom end of the oesophagus. It can be caused by vomiting. The patient will typically present with bright red haematemesis. The tear will usually heal by itself very quickly, though patients presenting with haematemesis will generally undergo endoscopy to check for other causes of bleeding.

Gastritis

This is inflammation of the stomach lining. It may present with dyspepsia, nausea and vomiting. Sometimes it may result in haematemesis and/or melaena. It can be caused by *H. pylori*; excessive consumption of alcohol, which can irritate the gastric lining; or by the use of non-steroidal anti-inflammatory drugs (NSAIDs) such as aspirin or ibuprofen. These drugs affect the way that the stomach can protect itself from the acid it produces. Stopping alcohol or NSAIDs may be enough to resolve gastritis. Otherwise PPI (see Table 4.1) drugs/*H. pylori* eradication may be prescribed (see below).

Helicobacter pylori (H. pylori)

This bacterium can exist in the stomach and has been found to cause gastritis, peptic ulceration and gastric cancers. It was not isolated until the 1980s (Warren and Marshall, 1983). It may be associated with functional dyspepsia. It manages to live in the stomach by neutralising the normally acidic environment surrounding it. Gastritis can occur as a result of this infection, as it impairs the mechanisms normally protecting the stomach mucosa. This can result in ulceration. Additionally the presence of *H. pylori* can lead to the stomach producing increased amounts of acid and so duodenal ulceration is more likely. Treatment of *H. pylori* consists of a combination of two or more antibiotics and a PPI tablet. This is known as triple or quadruple eradication therapy.

If not treated, *H. pylori* are thought to remain in the stomach for life. The bacterium is believed to be transmitted by the faecal–oral route, often during childhood. It is more prevalent in developing countries and its prevalence in developed countries is increased in those aged 55 and above. These differences are believed to be due to improvements in hygiene practices in the Western World (Brown, 2000).

H. pylori can be detected by a blood test called serology, which shows whether the body has produced antibodies to the bacterium. This test is best for when patients first present with dyspepsia. However, it is not effective for testing whether *H. pylori* has been successfully eradicated as even after eradication the body will continue to produce antibodies to the bacterium.

A good test for checking eradication is a urease breath test. The patient drinks a solution of urea which contains labelled carbon 13 or 14. *H. pylori* produces urease, which breaks down the urea to form carbon dioxide. The labelled carbon atoms can then be detected on the breath and a diagnosis of active *H. pylori* infection can be made.

An additional test is a stool antigen test. This detects the presence of the *H. pylori* antigen in the stool. It can show whether the *H. pylori* is present and, because it tests specifically for the antigen, can show whether the bacteria has been successfully eradicated or not.

Table 4.1 Common medications used for treating upper GI complaints.

Family of drugs	How they work	Names
Antacids	These drugs are salts which neutralise the gastric acid	Sodium bicarbonate Aluminium hydroxide Magnesium carbonate Magnesium trisilicate Calcium carbonate
Alginates	These act as an antacid and form a raft on top of the stomach contents. This reduces reflux and protects the oesophageal mucosa	Gaviscon Peptac
Histamine H2 receptors	These drugs block the action of histamine on receptors in stomach acid producing cells. Histamine acts on the stomach cells to cause acid production. By blocking its action, acid production is reduced	Cimetidine Ranitidine Famotidine Nizatidine
Proton pump inhibitors (PPIs)	These drugs work by blocking the proton pump in stomach acid-producing cells. They reduce acid production in the stomach considerably and are the most effective means of tackling symptoms caused by gastric acid. They are however relatively expensive	Omeprazole Lansoprazole Pantoprazole Rabeprazole Esomeprzole
Anti-emetics/ prokinetics	These drugs act on dopamine receptors in the brain. They also increase the rate of gastric emptying and increase peristalsis.	Domperidone Metaclopramide

The best tests for *H. pylori* are those involving taking biopsies from the stomach. A Rapid Urease Test can be performed at the time of an endoscopy. A biopsy is taken from the stomach and placed into a yellow medium containing urea and a pH indicator. If *H. pylori* are present then the urease it produces will turn the urea into ammonia and so raise the pH, turning the indicator red. The advantage of this test is that a diagnosis of *H. pylori* can be made at the time of the endoscopy, and any treatment can be initiated straight away. The most reliable way of diagnosing *H. pylori*, however, is to look for it in biopsies under the microscope. This has to be carried out by histopathologists and involves extensive preparation and staining of the biopsy. Consequently it may take a number of days before the presence of *H. pylori* can be confirmed.

Peptic ulcers

Peptic ulcers occur when areas of the mucosa in the oesophagus, stomach or duodenum break down or are eroded. Such areas are referred to as ulcers when they are larger than 0.5 cm. Smaller areas of ulceration are called erosions. Oesophageal ulcers have been dealt with in the gastro-oesophageal reflux section. In this section we will examine gastric and duodenal ulcers.

Gastric ulcers are more commonly seen in the elderly. Symptoms may include epigastric pain, often associated with food, as well as nausea, heartburn, anorexia and weight loss. Haematemesis and melaena may occur. Additionally anaemia may result due to blood loss from the ulcers. Some gastric ulcers can be cancerous; therefore when they are found on endoscopy they are biopsied and a repeat endoscopy is performed six weeks later following treatment to ensure that they are fully healed and are not cancerous.

Duodenal ulcers may present with symptoms of epigastric pain which may often be worse when hungry and relieved by food. Duodenal ulcers are rarely cancerous.

Peptic ulcers are often associated with *H. pylori*, though other factors such as NSAID use, smoking, stress and genetics may be contributory. Peptic ulcers can erode into a blood vessel, causing massive blood loss. They can also perforate, leading to contamination of the peritoneal cavity. This may lead to peritonitis and

---

Box 4.2 Lifestyle advice to offer people with dyspepsia symptoms

- There is little evidence available to show that lifestyle changes are effective in reducing the symptoms of dyspepsia. However, as many of the lifestyle changes may improve health in other ways it is worth encouraging patients to consider them.
- There may be a link between obesity and reflux symptoms. Advising sufferers to lose weight may help their reflux symptoms and reduce their chances of suffering with heart disease and some cancers.
- Smoking, alcohol, chocolate and fatty foods may all cause dyspepsia. Lifestyle advice around these areas may be helpful to dyspepsia patients.
- Eating large meals close to bedtime may precipitate dyspepsia symptoms. Patients should be encouraged to eat large meals at least three hours before going to bed, to allow the stomach to empty and so reduce reflux of gastric contents.

can be fatal. Ulcers may also cause gastric outlet obstruction. Such patients may present with persistent vomiting.

Though upper GI endoscopy is the first line of investigation, many patients with simple dyspepsia symptoms can be tested for *H. pylori* and receive eradication treatment if necessary, which will usually help ulcers to heal. This is called 'Test and Treat'. If symptoms continue in spite of confirmed eradication then endoscopy may be necessary. Refer to Box 4.2 regarding lifestyle advice to offer patients with dyspepsia symptoms.

Zollinger–Ellison syndrome

Zollinger–Ellison syndrome involves a tumour in the pancreas which secretes gastrin, causing the stomach to produce large amounts of acid. Patients may present with pain and multiple duodenal ulcers which do not respond to usual treatment. Additionally patients may have diarrhoea and steatorrhoea (pale, foul smelling, fatty stools which may often float in the toilet). The condition is diagnosed by measuring the amount of gastrin in the blood. A CT scan may reveal the presence of a pancreatic tumour. Very large doses of PPIs may be necessary to allow the ulceration to heal. Sometimes surgery can be performed to remove the tumour.

Care planning and nursing interventions

Nursing interventions for upper GI complaints consist initially (particularly in patients with symptoms of a GI bleed) of ensuring that the patient is haemodynamically stable by taking adequate observations and initiating management such as intravenous fluids and blood transfusions if required. When patients are suffering with nausea and vomiting, vomit bowls and tissues should be provided and changed as necessary. Medications prescribed to relieve the vomiting may be administered as appropriate. These can be given orally, but if the symptoms are severe, preparations designed to be given rectally, intramuscularly or intravenously may be administered. Patients may be anxious about their condition. Additionally they may have anxiety about the investigations they may have to undergo.

Some patients will require investigation; often upper GI endoscopy. Patients need to be physically prepared for the procedure, including remaining nil by mouth; however, it is important that patients are helped to understand the risks and benefits of the procedure to help them in the consent process. As well as being anxious about their condition, patients may have worries about undergoing invasive tests such as upper GI endoscopy; discussion with the nurse may well be a source of comfort and reassurance in these circumstances.

Following endoscopy, patients may be sedated and so should be closely monitored, including assessing conscious state, oxygen saturations, pulse and blood pressure. Once patients have recovered from the procedure, it is important that they are helped to understand the results of the procedure and the management plan for their condition.

Patients with upper GI complaints may require a variety of medications in conjunction with lifestyle changes. A key component of nursing care is helping patients to understand the medications they need to take and ensuring that they are able to comply with the treatment prescribed. The onset of upper GI symptoms may often be an ideal opportunity to identify lifestyle changes that could help relieve these symptoms. As these changes are part of a healthier lifestyle, this acute episode, when the patient is focused on their health, may be a good occasion to encourage adoption of them.

Activity: Nursing care scenario

Mrs Patricia Gladsone, a 78-year-old lady is admitted on to your ward. She has been having coffee ground vomitus and is passing melaena. She lives alone, although she does have a cat. She has been diagnosed with arthritis in the past and takes ibuprofen. Otherwise she has no health problems and is normally healthy. She does her own shopping and housework. She is widowed and has one son who lives about forty miles away.

- What may be the cause of this lady's symptoms?
- What nursing observations should be carried out for this lady?
- What investigations may this lady undergo?
- What nursing interventions will you need to carry out for this lady?
- List the concerns this lady may have.

Summary

In this chapter conditions of the upper GI tract have been considered. It was noted that there are a variety of upper GI complaints, with the vast majority of symptoms falling within the spectrum of dyspepsia. This can indicate anything from functional problems, where there is no actual organic disease process taking place, to cancer. Consequently there are guidelines (NICE, 2004) (Table 4.1) that provide guidance on how these patients should be managed. Nursing care may involve looking after the shocked patient suffering with an acute GI bleed through to the chronic symptoms of abdominal pain and nausea and vomiting. Knowledge of the various investigations that such patients may undergo is necessary for the nurse working in gastroenterology. Additionally, an understanding of the various medications and their modes of operation is essential. However, it is important that the opportunity of advocating lifestyle measures that may both relieve symptoms and reduce risks of other disease is taken when appropriate.

References

Ackroyd, M., Wakefield, S. E., Williams, J. L., Stoddard, C. J. and Reed, M. W. (1997) Surveillance of Barrett's esophagus: a need for guidelines? *Disease of the Esophagus*, **10**(3), 185–9.

British Society of Gastroenterology (2002) *Guidelines for the Management of Dyspepsia.* BSG, London.

British Society of Gastroenterology (2005) *Guidelines for the Diagnosis and Management of Barrett's Columnar Lined Oesophagus.* A report of the Working Party of the British Society of Gastroenterology. BSG, London. http://www.bsg.org.uk/images/stories/docs/clinical/guidelines/oesophageal/Barretts_Oes.pdf (accessed February 2011).

British Society of Gastroenterology (2006) *Guidelines on Complications of Gastrointestinal Endoscopy.* http://www.bsg.org.uk/clinical-guidelines/endoscopy/guidelines-on-complications-of-gastrointestinal-endoscopy.html (accessed February 2011).

Brown, L. M. (2000) *Helicobacter pylori*: epidemiology and routes of transmission. *Epidemiologic Reviews*, **22**(2), 283–97.

Cancer Research UK (2007) *Stomach Cancer UK.* http://publications.cancerresearchuk.org/epages/crukstore.sf/en_GB/?ObjectPath=/Shops/crukstore/Products/CSSTO07 (accessed February 2011).

Cancer Research UK (2009) *Cancerstats: Oesophageal Cancer.* http://info.cancerresearchuk.org/cancerstats/types/oesophagus/incidence/ (accessed February 2011).

Caygill, C. P., Watson, A., Lao-Sirieix, P. and Fitzgerald, R. C. (2004) Barrett's oesophagus and adenocarcinoma. *World Journal of Surgical Oncology*, **2**(12), 1–21.

Fitzgerald, R. (2005) Barrett's oesophagus: a clinical overview. *Gastrointestinal Nursing*, **3**(7), 27–33.

Forgacs, I. and Loganayagam, A. (2008) Editorial: overprescribing proton pump inhibitors. *British Medical Journal*, **336**(7634), 2–3.

Moayyedi, P., Shelley, S., Deeks, J. J., Delaney, B., Innes, M. and Forman, D. (2009) *Pharmacological Interventions for Non Ulcer Dyspepsia (Review).* The Cochrane Collaboration, Cochrane Library, Issue 1. http://onlinelibrary.wiley.com/o/cochrane/clsysrev/articles/rel0003/CD001960/pdf_fs.html (accessed February 2011).

National Institute for Health and Clinical Excellence (NICE) (2004) Dyspepsia – Management of dyspepsia in adults in primary care. http://guidance.nice.org.uk/CG17/Guidance/pdf/English (accessed February 2011).

Royal College of Anaesthetists (2001) *Implementing and Ensuring Safe Sedation Practice for Healthcare Procedures in Adults.* http://www.rcoa.ac.uk/docs/safesedationpractice.pdf (accessed February 2011).

Warren, J. R. and Marshall, B. (1983) Unidentified curved bacilli on gastric epithelium in active chronic gastritis (Letter). *Lancet*, 1983, **1**, 1273–5.

CHAPTER 5

Lower gastrointestinal complaints

Carol L. Cox

Introduction

In this chapter the following conditions will be considered: constipation, diarrhoea, wind and bloating, rectal pain and bleeding, mesenteric ischaemia, perforation, appendicitis, occult gastrointestinal (GI) bleeding, intestinal obstruction, intra-abdominal abscesses and pancreatitis. Each condition will be defined in association with its epidemiology and pathophysiology. Its assessment, diagnosis and associated care planning with nursing interventions will be discussed. At the conclusion of the chapter key points will be presented to assist you in caring for patients with lower GI complaints. It is essential that you become familiar with the anatomy and physiology of the GI tract in order to provide appropriate assessment, diagnosis of problems and care to patients with lower GI complaints.

The GI tract is remarkably efficient. Within approximately 4 hours of food being taken in the GI tract extracts nutrients from the food, processes them into the circulatory system and prepares leftover material for evacuation. The substances pass through 6 metres or more of intestine before being stored temporarily in the colon. In the colon water is removed and the remainder (faeces) is evacuated through the bowel, usually within a day or two. It is important to consider that when this system is compromised significant health problems can arise – some of them life-threatening.

By reading this chapter and carrying out the proposed activities you should achieve the following learning outcomes:

- Improve your knowledge of lower GI conditions
- Understand the management options available in treating lower GI conditions
- Discuss the nursing care required when managing lower GI conditions.

Constipation

Depending on a person's diet, age and daily activities, opening of the bowels (regularity) can be anything from three bowel movements a day to one every three days normally (Cox and Steggall, 2009; Marieb, 2003). The longer faecal material remains in the colon, the harder the faeces become and the more difficult it is to pass. A normal stool should not be either unusually hard or soft. People should not have to strain when defecating.

Epidemiology and pathophysiology

The causes of constipation vary (Crumbie, 1999). A busy lifestyle has been regarded as a contributing factor for most cases of constipation. This includes not taking or having the time to eat and drink properly, such as not eating enough fibre or drinking enough water (Swartz, 2006). In addition, not getting enough exercise and not taking the time to respond to an unmistakable urge to defecate are contributing factors. Research has found that emotional and psychological problems can contribute to the problem (NDDIC, 2007). However, chronic constipation may be a symptom of more serious conditions, such as irritable bowel syndrome (IBS), colorectal cancer, diabetes, Parkinson's disease, multiple sclerosis, an under-active thyroid gland and depression (NDDIC, 2007).

As individuals age, their bowel habits tend to vary from when they were younger (Bethel, 2008). For example, bottle-fed infants tend to have firmer stools and more bouts of constipation than breast-fed infants. Early on in life, some children develop a habit of 'holding on to their stool', and therefore become constipated when they start school or other activities because they are embarrassed to ask permission to use the toilet (Cox and Lee, 2010; Barnes, 2003). Toddlers often become constipated during toilet training if they are unwilling or afraid to use the toilet. Children may also avoid going to the toilet if they have splits or tears in their anus from straining at stool or other irritations (Cox and Lee; 2010; Barnes, 2003). Older people tend to develop constipation as they lose their thirst drive and subsequently do not drink enough liquid during the day (Cox, 2010). Individuals who are sedentary also develop constipation due to lack of exercise. Finally, some medications cause constipation. For example, narcotic-type medications used to treat pain such as codeine, iron supplements and some medicines used to control hypertension frequently lead to constipation developing when they are used for more than a few days.

Care planning and nursing interventions

Encourage patients to drink up to two litres of water a day. Reviewing a patient's medication regimen is helpful when it is suspect that the problem may be related to prescribed or over-the-counter medications. Health education/health promotion activities in which information is provided about nutrition and the need for fibre in diets can help patients make healthy choices regarding food consumption. Children that 'hold on to their stool', have a fear of going to the toilet or strain at stool should be referred to their GP for review and possible referral (Cox and Lee, 2010).

> **Activity**
> Consider the nursing care required for a patient complaining of constipation. Outline the factors that are most important to teach them about managing their care.

Diarrhoea

Diarrhoea is the passing of loose stools equating to more than 300 g in 24 hours in an adult (Lewis and Heaton, 1997). It is frequently caused by a virus or bacteria and can be acute (short term) or chronic (long term) (Marieb and Hoehn, 2007; Marieb, 2003). Chronic diarrhoea is the passing of loose stools for more than two to three weeks. The majority of people experience diarrhoea at some time in their lives. Symptoms frequently include stomach pains, nausea and vomiting. Symptoms may also include cold sweats and bloody stools.

Epidemiology and pathophysiology

The causes of diarrhoea are varied. It is generally related to the consumption of water contaminated with bacteria or food such as undercooked meat and eggs or inadequate kitchen hygiene. Box 5.1 indicates the primary causes of diarrhoea.

> **Box 5.1 Primary causes of diarrhoea**
> Diarrhoea is primarily caused by bacterial and viral infections and food poisoning. It can also be caused by bacteria or viruses that have been transmitted from person to person. It is important for people to wash their hands with soap and water after using the toilet and before preparing food or consuming food (Talley and O'Connor, 2006; Crumbie, 1999).

Diarrhoea occurs when micro-organisms irritate the mucous membrane of the gut, resulting in reabsorption of water into the small and large intestine. Certain types of bacteria, such as staphylococci, irritate the bowel by producing toxins. The irritated gut reacts by increasing peristalsis. It contracts excessively and irregularly. Hand hygiene is essential. People with dermatitis on their hands should not prepare food for others.

Antibiotics can cause some people to suffer with diarrhoea. The diarrhoea may continue for some time after the antibiotic course has been completed. The antibiotic alters the intestinal bacterial flora. The diarrhoea may continue until the flora recover. It is important to note this is not an allergic reaction to the antibiotic. Diarrhoea can also be caused by pseudomembranous colitis due to *Clostridium difficile* (*C. diff*), which may require hospitalisation. *C. diff* has been a troublesome problem for patients in hospital. It is an infection that can occur within two months of taking antibiotics or within a short time of being admitted to hospital. Several outbreaks have occurred over the past few years. It is a particular risk for children and the elderly.

Diarrhoea normally lasts for a few hours to a couple of days (Talley and O'Connor, 2006; Lewis and Heaton, 1997). Research indicates that although accidents are the leading cause of death amongst children in the developed world, diarrhoea accounted for 18% of the 10.6 million annual deaths of children under the age of five globally (Bryce *et al.* and the World Health Organization, 2005, cited in Bethel, 2008). This is mainly due to poor quality drinking water and malnutrition. There are also instances of people suffering with chronic diarrhoea. Table 5.1 lists the disorders that may cause chronic diarrhoea and Table 5.2 lists

Table 5.1 Causes of chronic diarrhoea (Duncan, 2011; Ellis and Cole, 2011; Goh *et al.*, 1996).

- Irritable bowel syndrome (IBS)
- Intolerance to gluten (wheat protein) or coeliac disease
- Acute, recurrent or chronic intestinal infections
- Chronic intestinal inflammation (ulcerative colitis and Crohn's disease)
- Chronic pancreatitis, which produces fatty stools
- Frequent use of laxatives
- Lactose intolerance
- Improper diet (consumption of too much alcohol, coffee or sweets)
- Metabolic disorders such as diabetes and thyrotoxicosis

Table 5.2 Symptoms of diarrhoea (McGrath, 2010; Bethel, 2008; Marieb and Hoehn, 2007).

- Frequent, watery motions
- Loss of appetite
- Nausea, vomiting
- Stomach pains
- Fever
- Dehydration

its symptoms. It should be noted that diarrhoea lasting more than three weeks is considered to be a chronic problem.

Care planning and nursing interventions

Patients should be encouraged in cases of acute diarrhoea to drink more fluids (3 to 4 litres a day). Liquids should contain sugar and salts. Ready-mixed rehydration sachets (e.g. Pedialyte, Dioralyte, Rehidrat) can be bought from the pharmacist and added to drinking water. Patients should be told that they should eat some foods containing salt – preferably soup due to its liquid content – and should eat normally as soon as their appetite returns.

In non-acute cases, encourage patients to maintain good standards of hygiene, washing their hands before and after handling food and after going to the toilet. Diarrhoea can be treated safely at home and usually subsides by itself within a few days to a week. Treatment with antibiotics is not required and may when taken by patients cause side-effects, such as chronic diarrhoea. Antidiarrhoeal agents, such as loperamide (e.g. Imodium), may be taken. Research has found that freeze-dried lactic acid bacteria does not prevent travellers' diarrhoea (Netdoctor, 2011).

Finally, nurses should provide guidance to patients who are travelling abroad. All drinking water should be boiled or consumed from sealed bottles. Salads should be avoided, as these may have been washed in unclean water. Encourage your patients to consume only vegetables that have been boiled or peeled and avoid ice-cream due to its bacterial content.

Activity

Describe the actions you think are critical to implement (in relation to infection control) to deter the spread of *Clostridium difficile*.

Wind and bloating

The gut usually contains about 200 ml of 'gas'. Every day a person passes 400–2000 ml of this gas out through their back passage as wind (or flatus, as it is technically known) (Marieb and Hoehn, 2007). Over 90% of flatus is made up of five gases. These are: nitrogen, oxygen, carbon dioxide, hydrogen and methane. The remaining 10% contains small amounts of other gases. Nitrogen and oxygen are derived from air which is swallowed. Carbon dioxide is produced by stomach acid mixing with bicarbonate in bile and pancreatic juices. These gases move into the small intestine, where most of the oxygen and carbon dioxide are absorbed into the blood stream. The nitrogen is passed into the colon (large bowel).

Epidemiology and pathophysiology

The small intestine is where food is digested and absorbed (Evers, 2008). Residue, such as dietary fibre and some carbohydrates, passes on to the colon. The colon contains bacteria that are essential for fermenting material that comes from the small intestine. The fermentation process produces large volumes of hydrogen, methane, carbon dioxide and other gases. Most of these gases are absorbed into the bloodstream through the intestinal wall and are eventually excreted in the breath (Evers, 2008). The remainder is passed as flatus. Table 5.3 lists the most frequent complaints associated with 'wind'. Each of these will be discussed in turn.

Table 5.3 Frequent complaints associated with wind (McGrath, 2010; Evers, 2008; Fry *et al.*, 2008).

Belching or burping (air eructation)
Chronic or repetitive burping (aerophagy)
Bloating
Rumblings/grumblings or noisy guts (borborygmi)

Belching or burping (air eructation)

When a person swallows, air passes into the stomach. A belch or burp is an involuntary expulsion of wind from the stomach when it becomes distended by swallowed air (Marieb, 2003). People who eat rapidly or gulp food and drink, drink lots of liquid with meals, chew gum, smoke or wear loose dentures are predisposed to swallowing air. Some people swallow their saliva to relieve heartburn. In these instances air is swallowed with the saliva. Other people swallow air without noticing it. This is especially true when people are nervous or tense. Fizzy drinks, including beer and sparkling wine, cause belching because they contain carbon dioxide which is released into the stomach.

Chronic or repetitive burping (aerophagy)

In this situation, air is not swallowed into the stomach. It is sucked into the gullet and rapidly expelled. Repetitive belching like this can last for several minutes and is embarrassing (Bickley and Szilagyi, 2007; Talley and O'Connor, 2006). There is no medical treatment. Its cure lies in realising the cause. Air cannot be sucked in when the jaws are separated, so repetitive belching can be temporarily controlled by clenching something like a pencil between the teeth.

Bloating

Bloating of the abdomen is frequently blamed on excess gas in the bowel. It is a common problem and generally experienced more acutely by women age 45 and above due to changes occurring in the GI tract (Swartz, 2006; Talley and O'Connor, 2006). Foods containing wheat become more difficult to digest. In people with irritable bowel syndrome (IBS), in which the intestine is more sensitive to distension, this is not the case. In IBS, normal amounts of gas cause discomfort. Because the muscular contractions of the gut are not coordinated, its contents do not move along in an orderly manner. Research has shown that when small amounts of gas are passed into the intestine, people with IBS experience bloating and pain, whereas other people tolerate the same or even larger amounts of gas without any discomfort. Bloating can also be caused by eating rich, fatty foods, which delay stomach emptying.

Abdominal distension is frequently seen in people who complain of bloating. This is normally related to relaxation of the abdominal muscles in an unconscious attempt to relieve the discomfort. The distension will usually disappear when the person lies down or contracts their abdominal muscles.

Rumblings/grumblings or noisy guts (borborygmi)

Bowel noises or borborygmi are produced when the liquid and gas contents of the intestine are shuffled backwards and forwards by peristalsis of the gut. The noises may be produced by hunger or anxiety, or when a person is frightened. Noises are common in IBS.

Crohn's disease and bowel obstruction can cause loud borborygmi. These conditions are associated with other symptoms such as severe abdominal pain and should be reported to a doctor (http://www.corecharity.org.uk/Windy-symptoms-Flatulence-belching-bloating-and-breaking-wind.html).

Care planning and nursing interventions

Treatment for bloating can be problematic. A high-fibre diet can cause bloating in some patients, but in other patients it relieves bloating. This is because fibre absorbs water in the intestines and gently distends it, which helps to prevent the uncoordinated contractions that are partly responsible for bloating. IBS may worsen when patients are stressed or anxious. Thus stress and anxiety may also be responsible for bloating. Recommending relaxation techniques can be useful for some patients. Administration of activated charcoal or a defoaming agent (containing simethicone) can help to reduce bloating. Recommending that patients avoid fizzy drinks may help as well. If the bloating is severe it may be necessary for the doctor or nurse, if an independent non-medical prescriber, to prescribe drugs that help to coordinate the contractions of the gut or prevent spasms.

Bloating due to a build up of gas also occurs in intestinal diseases like coeliac disease, Crohn's disease or bowel cancer. These conditions cause other symptoms such as weight loss, abdominal pain and diarrhoea. Each requires prompt medical investigation.

Activity

Identify the types of relaxation techniques that you could recommend to patients complaining of bloating.

Rectal pain and bleeding

Epidemiology and pathophysiology

Rectal pain is a common problem that many people have experienced. It usually appears as a mild discomfort, but on occasion the pain can be incapacitating because it is so painful. There are many causes of rectal pain. Most of these are not serious. Common causes of rectal pain are shown in Table 5.4. Table 5.5 shows less frequent causes of rectal pain.

Care planning and nursing interventions

Generally rectal pain does not require a visit to a Walk-in Centre or Accident & Emergency Department. Patients should be advised to contact their GP before going to the Walk-in Centre or hospital. However, an urgent referral to A&E may be required if the following conditions develop:

Table 5.4 Common causes of rectal pain (Hibberts, 2010/2011).

Haemorrhoids	Enlargement of a vein or veins at the anus; usually caused by straining during defecation
Anal fissure	A small tear in the skin at the opening of the rectum; usually caused when hard stool is passed
Proctalgia fugax	A condition associated with fleeting rectal pain and is more common in women and people under the age of 45
Levator ani syndrome	A syndrome that affects 6% of the US population and occurs in women slightly more often than in men; caused by spasm of the levator ani muscles

Table 5.5 Less frequent causes of rectal pain (Duncan, 2011; Ellis and Cole, 2011).

- Cancer
- Infection, including anorectal abscesses (proctitis)
- Inflammatory bowel disease (IBD) such as ulcerative colitis and Crohn's disease
- Foreign bodies in the rectum or rectal prolapse

- Rectal pain becomes more severe; particularly associated with fever and infectious discharge from the rectum
- Pain is no longer confined to the rectum but spreads to the abdomen
- The patient notices an increasing amount of rectal bleeding or a large amount of bleeding in one episode
- The patient thinks they have a foreign body in their rectum or suspect rectal prolapse is the cause of pain (http://www.emedicinehealth.com/rectal_pain/page3_em.htm)

Activity
Your patient notices a large amount of rectal bleeding each time they open their bowels. Articulate the advice you should give to this patient.

Mesenteric ischaemia

Acute mesenteric ischaemia is a relatively rare disorder that is a potentially fatal vascular emergency (Prather, 2007; Oldenburg *et al.*, 2004). It has an overall mortality rate of 60% to 80% (Oldenburg *et al.*, 2004). Nonspecific clinical findings and limitations inherent in diagnostic studies make the diagnosis difficult to discern. A delay in diagnosis leads to increased mortality rates. Mesenteric ischaemia is caused by a decreased intestinal blood flow that is associated with a number of mechanisms. Decreased intestinal blood flow results in ischaemia and reperfusion damage at the cellular level that can progress to the development of mucosal injury, tissue necrosis, and metabolic acidosis (Prather *et al.*, 2007; Oldenburg *et al.*, 2004).

Epidemiology and pathophysiology

Seventy per cent of mesenteric blood flow is directed to the mucosal and submucosal layers of the bowel with the remaining being directed to the directed to the muscularis and serosal layers of the bowel (Oldenburg *et al.*, 2004). The intestine has substantial collateral circulation that does allow for some protection from ischaemia. It is able to compensate for approximately a 75% acute reduction in mesenteric blood flow for up to 12 hours, without substantial injury (Prather, 2007; Oldenburg *et al.*, 2004). Survival from mesenteric ischaemia is 50% if the problem is identified within 24 hours of the onset of symptoms (Oldenburg *et al.*, 2004). It drops to 30% if diagnosis is delayed beyond 24 hours (Oldenburg *et al.*, 2004).

Intestinal ischaemia can be divided into arterial and venous aetiologies. It can be either acute or chronic. The majority of ischaemias are secondary to arterial causes. Every disease and condition that affects the arteries, including atherosclerosis, arteritis, aneurysms, arterial infections, dissections, arterial emboli and thrombosis occur in the intestinal arteries. Table 5.6 shows the further divisions of acute mesenteric ischaemia (AMI).

Chronic mesenteric ischaemia (CMI) generally results from longstanding atherosclerotic disease of two or more mesenteric vessels. Other nonatheromatous causes of chronic mesenteric ischaemia involve vasculitides such as Takayasu arteritis. Symptoms of chronic mesenteric ischaemia derive from the gradual reduction in blood flow to the intestine that occurs during eating. The intake of food increases total blood flow to the intestine by as much as 15%. A rare cause of

Table 5.6 Further divisions of acute mesenteric ischaemia (AMI) (Prather, 2007; Oldenburg *et al.*, 2004; Howard *et al.*, 1996).

- Arterial embolism
- Arterial thrombosis
- Nonocclusive aetiology

chronic mesenteric ischaemia is related to coeliac artery compression syndrome (CACS). CACS entails external compression of the coeliac artery by the median arcuate ligament or the coeliac ganglion (Howard *et al.*, 1996).

As previously indicated, mortality rates are high and range from 60–100% depending on the source of obstruction in chronic cases (Oldenburg *et al.*, 2004; Howard *et al.*, 1996). Early and aggressive diagnosis and treatment has been shown to significantly decrease the mortality rate if the diagnosis is made prior to the development of peritonitis.

Age is a factor in the development of mesenteric ischaemia. It is generally a disease of the older population, with the usual age of onset being older than 60 years, although with other predisposing risk factors it may be seen in younger patients. Clinical presentation is largely dependent on the underlying aetiology, with acute mesenteric ischaemia (AMI) and chronic mesenteric ischaemia (CMI) presenting differently. In acute mesenteric ischaemia the patient experiences severe poorly localised abdominal pain with minimal abdominal examination findings but with a history of risk factors. Usually the onset of pain is gradual. It may be refractory to opioid analgesics and prior episodes of pain, frequently related to meals, known as intestinal angina, may have been experienced. Nausea and vomiting are frequently present, and diarrhoea may occur in as many as 50% of patients. Chronic mesenteric ischaemia causes postprandial (after eating) abdominal pain and weight loss. The pain is chronic and dull as the obstructive process worsens. Some patients with chronic mesenteric ischaemia may experience sitophobia (fear of eating).

Care planning and nursing interventions

In suspected cases of mesenteric ischaemia prompt referral to an Accident & Emergency Department is imperative. Nurses should suspect mesenteric ischaemia in older patients complaining of poorly localised abdominal pain, postprandial episodes of pain and weight loss.

Activity
Identify the presenting factors associated with acute and chronic mesenteric ischaemia.

Perforation

Perforations of the GI tract are rare (Goh *et al.*, 2006). However, when they occur they are a dangerous complication leading to peritonitis and even death from septicaemia. Perforations may be seen in the oesophagus, stomach or in the intestines, including the rectum (Don and Rockey, 1999). Certain investigative procedures, such as endoscopy may cause a perforation (Goh *et al.*, 2006). In this instance, the endoscope pierces the wall of the bowel. Polypectomies may also result in perforation at the site of the polyp removal.

Epidemiology and pathophysiology

The signs and symptoms of GI perforations vary and generally depend on the type and timing of the perforation (Goh *et al.*, 2006). Patients with a colonic perforation will experience severe abdominal pain and a have a rigid abdomen and demonstrate guarding of the abdomen within 24 hours of the procedure (Don and Rockey, 1999). There have been instances where it has taken up to a week to ten days for symptoms to develop. Perforation should be suspected when patients demonstrate rebound tenderness (a symptom of peritonitis) following a colonoscopy (Fry *et al.*, 2008). It will be diagnosed by abdominal X-ray, in which free air is seen in the abdomen, computed tomography (CT) or a gastrograffin swallow done under fluoroscopy (Don and Rockey, 1999). Tiny perforations in well-prepared bowels may close on their own when antibiotics are administered in association with conservative treatment of bowel rest. Serial abdominal examinations are essential to discern deterioration. Large perforations require surgical repair.

Care planning and nursing interventions

The nurse must be vigilant when evaluating patients who complain of excessive pain, do not experience pain relief with passing flatus, or who develop pain hours after an endoscopy. Therefore the nurse or technician must watch the patient closely during and after the procedure to assure that the patient is stable and comfortable when discharged. The nurse should check the patient for pyrexia, tachycardia and elevated white blood cells. In addition to being vigilant in evaluating patients' complaints of abdominal pain after an endoscopy, the nurse should question patients as to whether they are experiencing any abdominal pain, fever or tachycardia when follow-up telephone calls are made 24 hours following the procedure. Patients should be kept nil by mouth following the procedure when there is a concern that the endoscopy has been complex. In addition, if patients have been administered throat spray then they should remain nil by mouth for at least one hour following the procedure to avoid aspiration. Nurses should bring the patient's complaints to the attention of the doctor as soon as possible.

Gastrointestinal nurse specialists will usually see perforations that are scope-related. However, they should be on guard to other triggers for this complication.

Patients may be followed for other GI complaints, such as Crohn's disease, diverticulitis, peptic ulcer, inflammatory bowel disease, cancer or toxic megacolon, in which a perforation may develop.

Activity

Refer to Chapter 9. Your patient has sustained an oesophageal perforation during endoscopy. Describe the emergency actions you should implement in this situation.

Appendicitis

Appendicitis is an inflammation of the appendix. The appendix is a closed-ended, narrow tube up to several inches in length that attaches to the caecum, which is the first part of the colon. The lining of the appendix produces mucus, which flows from the appendix into the caecum. The appendix's inner wall contains lymphatic tissue, which forms part of the immune system that produces antibodies (Marieb and Hoehn, 2007). Therefore it is thought that the appendix has a role in preventing infection from developing in the colon.

Epidemiology and pathophysiology

Appendicitis occurs when the opening from the appendix into the caecum becomes blocked. This blockage may be due to a build-up of thick mucus within the appendix or to stool that enters the appendix from the caecum. The mucus or stool hardens (fecalith) and then blocks the opening (Marieb and Hoehn, 2007; Marieb, 2003). In other cases, the lymphatic tissue in the appendix may swell and block the opening of the appendix which means the mucus can't be excreted from the appendix into the colon. Once the blockage occurs, bacteria which normally are found in the appendix begin to invade (infect) the wall of the appendix causing an inflammation. It is possible for the appendix to rupture from the inflammation and distension caused by the infection. If left untreated, the infection can spread throughout the abdomen. Generally the infection is confined to a small area surrounding the appendix forming a peri-appendiceal abscess.

Sometimes appendicitis will heal without surgical treatment. This can occur when the infection and inflammation do not spread throughout the abdomen. In this case, pain and other inflammatory symptoms may disappear. This can occur in elderly patients and when antibiotics are used. Some time later, the patients may, when being examined by their GP for some other complaint, have a lump or mass in the right lower abdomen. This is due to the scarring that occurs during the healing process. The lump or mass may raise a suspicion of cancer.

Perforation is the most frequent complication of appendicitis. Subsequent to perforation, a peri-appendiceal abscess, which is a collection of infected pus, or diffuse peritonitis, which is an infection of the entire lining of the abdomen and the pelvis, can occur (Swartz, 2006). The major reason for an appendiceal perforation is delay in diagnosis and treatment. The longer the delay the more likely it is that a perforation may occur. The risk of perforation 36 hours after the onset of symptoms is at least 15%. Therefore, once appendicitis has been confirmed, surgery should be done without delay.

Blockage of the intestine is a less common complication of appendicitis. It occurs when the inflammation surrounding the appendix causes the development of a paralytic ileus; peristalsis stops. Above the blockage, the intestine fills with liquid and gas. Abdominal distension ensues and nausea and vomiting may occur. A feared complication of appendicitis is sepsis.

Appendicitis is diagnosed by history, physical examination (positive obdurator, psoas or Rofsing sign), elevated temperature, elevated white blood cell count, abdominal X-ray, (showing red blood cells), ultrasound, barium enema, computed tomography (CT) Scan and laparoscopy (Edie, 2010; McGrath, 2010; Swartz, 2006). There is no single test that will diagnose appendicitis with certainty. The approach to suspected appendicitis may include a period of observation, the tests listed in this chapter and exploratory surgery.

Care planning and nursing interventions
As the main symptom of appendicitis is abdominal pain nurses should observe for its location. In early stages of appendicitis, patients will indicate that the pain is initially poorly localised. When asked about their pain they will point with their finger in a circular motion indicating that it is somewhere around the central part of their abdomen. Pain that is poorly localised is confined to the small intestine or colon, including the appendix. Another common, early symptom of appendicitis is loss of appetite, which may progress to nausea and even vomiting. However, nausea and vomiting also occur in later stages due to intestinal obstruction. Therefore nurses should be cognisant of this complication. It may be necessary to pass a nasogastric tube to drain the contents of the stomach and intestine. When surgical intervention is required, post-operative nursing care should be provided according to the protocol of the healthcare institution where the nurse is working.

> **Activity**
> Explain the nursing observations you will undertake when a patient is suspected of having appendicitis.

Occult gastrointestinal bleeding

The most common form of GI bleeding is occult GI bleeding. Its causes are many. GI bleeding usually presents as either iron deficiency anaemia or faecal occult blood (Green and Rockey, 2004; Bini *et al.*, 1999). These types of bleeding are unrecognised by the patient, and therefore are termed 'occult' bleeding.

Epidemiology and pathophysiology

Iron deficiency anaemia results from chronic blood loss. It is the most common form of anaemia. It is seen in children and women of child-bearing age and pregnant women. It is common in women during their reproductive years because of menstrual and pregnancy-associated blood losses (Green and Rockey, 2004). In men and postmenopausal women that present with iron deficiency anaemia the most common cause is GI tract pathology resulting in blood loss. Obscure GI bleeding refers to bleeding that the patient readily observes. It is generated from a lesion in the GI tract that may be difficult to identify. Frequently it appears to emanate from the small bowel.

In order for blood to present in stool, approximately 150 to 200 mL of blood must be in the stomach (Swartz, 2006). Blood which presents in the stool is termed melaena and may be seen as black tarry stools that have an unpleasant odour. Patients with gastroduodenal bleeding of up to 100 mL per day may have normal-appearing stools. Occult bleeding is generally identified by a faecal occult blood test (FOBt) (Bini *et al.*, 1999). In the UK, all people over the age of 60 are invited to undertake a FOBt to rule out occult GI bleeding associated with bowel cancer. If bleeding occurs over a long period of time, it may present as iron depletion and anaemia.

Iron deficiency anaemia

Iron deficiency anaemia is defined by the presence of anaemia and low iron stores. The diagnosis of iron deficiency and iron deficiency anaemia should be suspected any time a low serum haemoglobin level or haematocrit is encountered (Rockey, 2005; Rockey, 1999). In addition, a reduced mean corpuscular volume (MCV) supports the diagnosis, but is not definitive. Iron deficiency anaemia is generally

Table 5.6 Causes of occult bleeding (Goh *et al.*, 2006; Rockey, 2005; Rockey, 1999).

- Colon cancer; especially lesions in the right colon

- Lesion (or lesions) from any location in the GI tract Lesion (or lesions) in the oral cavity or nasopharyngeal area

- Ulcerations in the upper GI tract such as oesophageal, gastric or duodenal ulcers

- The most common cause of iron deficiency anaemia worldwide is probably hookworm (http://www.cdc.gov/NCIDOD/dpd/parasites/hookworm/factsht_hookworm.htm). These small parasites can remove significant amounts of blood from the colon on an ongoing basis if left untreated

confirmed by a low serum ferritin level in the setting of anaemia (Hgb less than 11.5 mg/dL for women and 12.5 for men). A very low ferritin level (less than 20 ng/mL) is essentially diagnostic of iron deficiency anaemia (Bini *et al.*, 1999). A diagnosis of iron deficiency anaemia in postmenopausal women or men will lead to extensive evaluation (Rockey *et al.*, 1993; Rockey *et al.*, 1998; Rockey *et al.*, 1999). In some instances, patients may have iron deficiency without anaemia, though by definition, anaemia will develop in the iron-deficient state as long as blood loss continues without iron replacement.

Care planning and nursing interventions
The standard approach to patients with iron deficiency anaemia is to directly evaluate the GI tract. This is most commonly done by examining the GI tract mucosa by endoscopy and colonoscopy. Oesophagogastroduodenoscopy endoscopic procedures may be performed under sedation or through a throat spray. The nurse must ensure that the patient's airway is maintained both during the procedure and following the procedure in recovery. In the colon a colonoscopy is the best test. Sometimes routine radiographic tests may be undertaken (barium enema, upper GI series). However, these tests have fallen out of favour and are infrequently used. Radiographic studies are effective for detecting masses and large ulcerating lesions, but are not very accurate at detecting mucosal lesions.

A newer technology in the area of small bowel imaging is capsule endoscopy (Cave, 2006; Iddan *et al.*, 2000). This involves the patient swallowing a capsule approximately 11×26 mm in size that contains a camera, two batteries and a radiofrequency transmitter. The capsule obtains at least two images per second. These images are transmitted to a recording device worn by the patient. The data are then downloaded to a computer workstation loaded with software that allows images to be analysed (Cave, 2006). Because of the capsule's small size, it passes harmlessly through the GI tract, typically within 24 hours, in nearly all patients. Patients will frequently question the nurse about the size of the capsule and express concern regarding its passage. In these instances patients should be reassured that they will not normally experience any discomfort in passing the capsule. A critical issue in assessing patients who may have iron deficiency anaemia is to appropriately correlate GI lesions with the degree of blood loss. Although it is evident that mass lesions and severe ulcerative upper GI lesions can lead to substantial blood loss (up to 20 mL per day), it is unlikely that small lesions and erosions (such as mild inflammation and especially small adenomas) will bleed enough to lead to iron deficiency (Looker *et al.*, 1997). Thus judgement must be used when linking GI tract lesions to iron deficiency anaemia.

Once a diagnosis of iron deficiency anaemia has been determined, iron therapy should be instituted. Oral ferrous sulfate is recommended. It is inexpensive and effective (the recommended dose is 300 mg/three times daily) in treating the disorder. In those who are intolerant to ferrous sulfate, ferrous gluconate or fumarate are acceptable alternatives. Parenteral iron therapy should be administered only to patients that have severe malabsorption syndrome or who are intolerant to iron supplements.

Activity
You suspect your patient may have iron deficiency anaemia. Describe the nursing actions you will take to confirm your suspicion.

Intestinal obstruction

Intestinal obstruction is generally evident by paralytic ileus, nausea, vomiting, elevated temperature and peritonitis (which may be acute and involve sepsis). Intestinal obstruction is a partial or complete blockage of the bowel that results in the failure of the intestinal contents to pass through (Evers, 2008; Fry *et al.*, 2008).

Epidemiology and pathophysiology

Obstruction of the bowel may be due to either a mechanical cause, such as an adhesion, or an ileus, which is a condition in which the peristaltic action of the bowel ceases. Paralytic ileus is also called pseudo-obstruction and is one of the major causes of intestinal obstruction in infants and children. Early signs of obstruction include abdominal distension, abdominal fullness, wind/gas, abdominal pain and cramping, faecal odour to the breath, constipation, diarrhoea, nausea and vomiting.

Table 5.7 Causes of paralytic ileus (Evers, 2008; Fry *et al.*, 2008).

- Chemical, electrolyte, or mineral disturbances (such as decreased potassium levels)
- Complications of intra-abdominal surgery
- Decreased blood supply to the abdominal area (mesenteric artery ischaemia)
- Injury to the abdominal blood supply
- Intra-abdominal infection
- Kidney or lung disease
- Use of certain medications, especially narcotics
- Bacterial, viral, or food poisoning (gastroenteritis), frequently seen in older children and may be associated with appendicitis

Table 5.8 Mechanical causes of intestinal obstruction (Evers, 2008; Fry *et al.*, 2008).

- Abnormal tissue growth
- Adhesions or scar tissue that form after surgery
- Foreign bodies (ingested materials that obstruct the intestines)
- Gallstones
- Hernias
- Impacted faeces (stool)
- Intussusception
- Tumors blocking the intestines
- Volvulus (twisted intestine)

Risk factors associated with necrosis include intestinal cancer, Crohn's disease, hernia and previous abdominal surgery. In the newborn infant, paralytic ileus that is associated with destruction of the bowel wall (necrotising enterocolitis) is life-threatening and may lead to blood and lung infections.

Diagnosing intestinal obstruction:
When listening to the abdomen with a stethoscope, high-pitched bowel sounds may be heard at the onset of mechanical obstruction. If the obstruction has persisted for some time or the bowel has been significantly damaged, bowel sounds will decrease and eventually become silent. Early paralytic ileus is determined by decreased or absent bowel sounds. Tests that will confirm an obstruction include an abdominal computed tomography (CT scan), abdominal X-ray, barium enema and upper GI and small bowel series (Edie, 2010).

Care planning and nursing interventions

The nurse should be prepared to pass a nasogastric (NG) tube into the stomach or intestine to relieve abdominal distension and vomiting. The patient should be prepared for surgery to relieve the obstruction if the tube does not relieve the symptoms, or if there are signs of tissue death. Patients experiencing a bowel obstruction will be in extreme discomfort and should be medicated appropriately to relieve pain. Medications to reduce anxiety should also be administered where appropriate. Close monitoring of intake and output are essential; particularly post-operatively. It is not uncommon for patients to develop anasarca post-operatively. Fluids should be managed carefully to avoid overload. Patients should be reassured that 'fluid in the tissues' or 'swelling of the tissues' will resolve.

Complications of intestinal obstruction that nurses should monitor for include electrolyte imbalances, infection, jaundice, perforation of the intestine, necrosis of tissue causing infection and gangrene. Risk factors associated with necrosis include intestinal cancer, Crohn's disease, hernia, and previous abdominal surgery. In the newborn infant, paralytic ileus that is associated with destruction of the bowel wall (necrotising enterocolitis) is life-threatening and may lead to blood and lung infections.

> **Activity**
> Explain the safety measures that should be undertaken when passing a NG tube and giving medicines through the tube. (You should check the hospital policy and procedure manual where you are practising regarding the passage of NG tubes and the administration of medicines through NG tubes if you have questions about this activity.)

Intra-abdominal abscesses

An intra-abdominal abscess is a pocket of infected fluid and pus located inside the abdominal cavity. There may be more than one abscess present. Symptoms associated with intra-abdominal abscesses, depending on their location, may include abdominal pain and distention, chills, diarrhoea, fever, anorexia, nausea and vomiting, feelings of fatigue and general weakness and rectal tenderness and fullness (Fry *et al.*, 2008; Prather, 2007).

Epidemiology and pathophysiology

Generally an intra-abdominal abscess is caused by a ruptured appendix, ruptured intestinal diverticulum, inflammatory bowel disease or parasite infection in the intestines (*Entamoeba histolytica*) (Fry *et al.*, 2008). However, it may be caused by other conditions such as pancreatitis. Risk factors associated with an intra-abdominal abscess include prior appendicitis, diverticulitis, perforated ulcer disease or surgery that may have infected the abdominal cavity.

Diagnosing an intra-abdominal abscess

Diagnosing an intra-abdominal abscess involves a full blood count (FBC). A FBC may show a higher than normal white blood cell count (WBC). Furthermore, a comprehensive metabolic panel may show liver, kidney or blood chemistry problems. A CT scan of the abdomen will show an intra-abdominal abscess. After the CT scan is done, a needle may be placed through the skin into the abscess cavity to confirm the diagnosis and treat the abscess. Abdominal X-rays and ultrasound scans of the abdomen may also be used in the diagnostic process. In some instances a laparotomy may be required to diagnose the condition.

Care planning and nursing interventions

Treatment requires the administration of intravenous antibiotics and drainage. The nurse may be called upon to assist in draining the abscess and is responsible for assessing drainage output and dressing changes. Drainage involves placing a needle through the skin into the abscess and the insertion of a drain or drains. This is generally done under X-ray guidance. The patient should be told that the drain or drains will be left in place for days or weeks until the abscess resolves. Strict measurement of drainage every 4 to 8 hours is required.

In some instances, abscesses cannot be safely drained via X-ray guidance. In such instances, a laparotomy must be performed. As a laparotomy normally requires the administration of general anaesthesia, patients should be monitored and recovered according to hospital post-operative procedures. Nurses should monitor for possible complications such as return of the abscess, rupture of an abscess, spread of the infection causing general peritonitis and sepsis.

Activity

Identify the important aspects of aseptic technique that nurses should employ when assisting with the drainage of an abscess or changing dressings on a patient's abdominal drain sites.

Pancreatitis

Pancreatitis is inflammation of the pancreas that occurs suddenly and usually resolves in a few days with treatment. The pancreas is a large gland behind the stomach and close to the duodenum which is the first part of the small intestine. The pancreas secretes digestive enzymes into the duodenum through the pancreatic duct. Pancreatic enzymes join with bile, which is a liquid produced in the liver and stored in the gallbladder. This liquid is used to digest food. The pancreas also releases the hormones insulin and glucagon into the bloodstream. These hormones help the body regulate the glucose it takes from food for energy. A serious complication of pancreatitis is sepsis (Russo *et al.*, 2004).

Epidemiology and pathophysiology

Normally, digestive enzymes secreted by the pancreas do not become active until they reach the small intestine (Marieb and Hoehn, 2007). But when the pancreas is inflamed, the enzymes inside it attack and damage the tissues that produce them. Pancreatitis can be either acute or chronic. Either form is serious and can lead to complications in which the patient becomes critically ill. In severe cases, infection and permanent tissue damage may occur as well as shock and death when there is bleeding in the pancreas. The usual cause of acute pancreatitis is gallstones (cholelithiasis), which cause inflammation in the pancreas as they pass through the common bile duct. Chronic alcoholism is also a common cause. Some other causes of acute pancreatitis are abdominal trauma, medications, infections, tumours, and genetic abnormalities of the pancreas. Both forms of pancreatitis occur more often in men than women (Russo *et al.*, 2004).

Chronic pancreatitis is an inflammation of the pancreas that does not heal or improve. Over time the inflammation worsens and permanent damage occurs. Chronic pancreatitis, like acute pancreatitis, occurs when digestive enzymes attack the pancreas and nearby tissues. The patient experiences episodes of acute pain. Chronic pancreatitis is normally seen in patients between the ages of 30 and 40 (Russo *et al.*, 2004). The most common cause of chronic pancreatitis is many years of heavy alcohol use.

Diagnosing pancreatitis

A comprehensive medical history and physical examination begin the process of determining pancreatitis (Swartz, 2006; Talley and O'Connor, 2006). Assessing for substance abuse (alcohol and drugs) is essential. Blood tests will be ordered to assist in the diagnosis. In acute pancreatitis, blood contains at least three times the normal amount of amylase and lipase, which are digestive enzymes formed

Table 5.9 Symptoms of acute pancreatitis (Talley and O'Connor, 2006; Russo *et al.*, 2004).

- Generally begins with gradual or sudden pain in the upper abdomen that sometimes extends to the back
- Pain may be mild at first and get worse after eating
- Pain is frequently severe and may become constant and last for several days
- Swollen and tender abdomen
- Nausea and vomiting
- Fever
- Tachycardia
- Dehydration and hypotension

Table 5.10 Symptoms of chronic pancreatitis (Talley and O'Connor, 2006; Russo *et al.*, 2004).

- Upper abdominal pain (although some patients experience no pain at all)
- Pain may spread to the back, feel worse when eating or drinking, and become constant and disabling. In some cases, abdominal pain goes away as the condition worsens, most likely because the pancreas is no longer making digestive enzymes.
- Nausea
- Vomiting
- Weight loss
- Diarrhoea
- Oily stools

Table 5.11 Causes of chronic pancreatitis (Swartz, 2006; Talley and O'Connor, 2006).

- Hereditary disorders of the pancreas (may present in people under the age of 30)
- Cystic fibrosis (the most common inherited disorder causing chronic pancreatitis)
- Hypercalcaemia
- Hyperlipidaemia or hypertriglyceridaemia
- Medications
- Some autoimmune disorders

in the pancreas. Changes may also be seen in blood components such as glucose, calcium, magnesium, sodium, potassium and bicarbonate. Diagnosing acute pancreatitis is frequently difficult because of the deep location of the pancreas (Russo *et al.*, 2004). In chronic pancreatitis, blood tests may reveal whether the pancreas is still making digestive enzymes. However, sometimes digestive enzymes will appear normal even though the patient has chronic pancreatitis. In the more advanced stages of chronic pancreatitis malabsorption and diabetes can occur. In these instances, blood, urine and stool tests will be ordered to help diagnose chronic pancreatitis and monitor its progression. For both acute and chronic pancreatitis one or more of the following tests will also be ordered: abdominal ultrasound, CT scan, endoscopic ultrasound (EUS) and magnetic resonance cholangiopancreatography (MRCP) (Edie, 2010).

Care planning and nursing interventions

Nurses should prepare the patient who is experiencing acute pancreatitis for a few days' stay in the hospital for the administration of intravenous (IV) fluids, antibiotics and medication to relieve pain. The patient must remain nil by mouth so that the pancreas can rest. If vomiting occurs, a nasogastric tube should be inserted to remove fluid and air. In severe cases, in which hospitalisation is protracted, the patient may be treated in an Intensive Care or High Dependency Unit. Special tube feedings may be administered for several weeks while the pancreas heals. Before leaving the hospital nurses should advise the patient not to smoke, drink alcoholic beverages or eat fatty meals. In chronic pancreatitis, when a normal diet is resumed synthetic pancreatic enzymes may be prescribed. Enzymes should be taken with every meal to help the patient digest food and regain weight. A diet that is low in fat and includes small, frequent meals should be planned through the assistance of a dietitian. Patients should be encouraged to drink a litre of fluid each day and limit or avoid caffeinated beverages.

Cholelithiasis that causes acute pancreatitis generally requires a cholecystectomy. If the pancreatitis is severe, stones may be removed via endoscopic retrograde cholangiopancreatography (ERCP). In these cases, when either sedation or a throat spray is used, close monitoring during recovery of the patient is essential to prevent aspiration.
When infection is present, ERCP may be employed to drain the infected area. A laparotomy may also be necessary to find sources of bleeding and to rule out conditions that resemble pancreatitis, or to remove severely damaged pancreatic tissue.

> ## Activity
> Write a nursing care plan for a patient who has acute pancreatitis.

Summary

In this chapter the following conditions have been considered: constipation, diarrhoea, wind and bloating, rectal pain and bleeding, mesenteric ischaemia, perforation, appendicitis, occult GI bleeding, intestinal obstruction, intra-abdominal abscesses and pancreatitis. Each condition was defined in association with its epidemiology and pathophysiology. Assessment, diagnosis and associated care planning with nursing interventions were also discussed. It has been indicated that knowledge of the anatomy and physiology of the GI tract is essential in assisting you to care for patients with lower GI complaints. Practical points have been shown in tables throughout the text to assist you in identifying causes and symptoms associated with each condition.

References

Barnes, K. (2003) Common paediatric problems. In *Paediatrics: A Clinical Guide For Nurse Practitioners* (ed. K. Barnes), Chapter 2. Butterworth-Heinemann, London.

Bethel, J. (2008) Abdominal and genitor-urinary illness. In: *Paediatric Minor Emergencies* (ed. J. Bethel), Chapter 20. M&K Update Ltd, Keswick, Cumbria.

Bickley, L. and Szilagyi, P. (2007) *Bates' Guide to Physical Examination*, 5th edn. Lippincott, Philadelphia.

Bini, E. J., Rajapaksa R. C. and Weinshel, E. H. (1999) The findings and impact of nonrehydrated guaiac examination of the rectum (FINGER) study: a comparison of 2 methods of screening for colorectal cancer in asymptomatic average-risk patients. *Archives of Internal Medicine*, **159**, 2022.

Cave, D. R. (2006) Technology insight: current status of video capsule endoscopy. *Nature Clinical Practice Gastroenterology & Hepatology*, **3**(3), 158–64.

Cox, C. (2010) Assessment of disability including care of the older adult. In: *Physical Assessment for Nurses*, 2nd edn (ed. C. Cox), Chapter 13. Wiley-Blackwell, Oxford.

Cox, C. and Lee, P. (2010) Assessment of the child. In: *Physical Assessment for Nurses*, 2nd edn (ed. C. Cox), Chapter 12. Wiley-Blackwell, Oxford.

Cox, C. and Steggall, M. (2009) A step-by-step guide to performing a complete abdominal examination. *Journal of Gastrointestinal Nursing*, **7**(1), 10–17.

Crumbie, A. (1999) The abdomen. In: *Nurse Practitioners: Clinical Skills and Professional Issues* (eds. M. Walsh, A. Crumbie and S. Reveley), Chapter 9. Butterworth-Heinemann, Oxford.

Don, C. and Rockey, M. D. (1999) Perforation of the gastrointestinal tract secondary to ingestion of foreign bodies. *New England Journal of Medicine*, **341**, 38–46.

Duncan, J. (2011) Nursing assessment in inflammatory bowel disease. *Gastrointestinal Nursing*, **9**(1), 14–20.

Edie, J. (2010) Imaging techniques. In: *Physical Assessment for Nurses*, 2nd edn (ed. C. Cox), Chapter 16. Oxford: Wiley-Blackwell.

Ellis, M. and Cole, A. (2011) Crohn's disease in children and adolescents. *Gastrointestinal Nursing*, **9**(1), 41–6.

Evers, B. M. (2008) Small intestine. In: *Sabiston Textbook of Surgery*, 18th edn (eds. C. M. Townsend, R. D. Beauchamp, B. M. Evers and K. L. Mattox), Chapter 48. W. B. Saunders, St Louis.

Fry, R. D., Mahmoud, N., Maron, D. J., Ross, H. M. and Rombeau, J. (2008) Colon and rectum. In: *Sabiston Textbook of Surgery*, 18th edn (eds. C. M. Townsend, R. D. Beauchamp, B. M. Evers and K. L. Mattox), Chapter 50. W. B. Saunders, St Louis.

Green, B. T. and Rockey, D. C. (2004) Gastrointestinal endoscopic evaluation of premenopausal women with iron deficiency anaemia. *Journal of Clinical Gastroenterology*, **38**, 104–9.

Goh, B. K., Chow, P. K., Quah, H. M., Ong, H. S., Eu, K. W., Ooi, L. L., Wong, W. K. and Fine, K. D. (1996) The prevalence of occult gastrointestinal bleeding in celiac sprue. *New England Journal of Medicine*, **334**, 1163–7.

Goh, B. K., Chow, P. K., Quah, H. M., Ong, H. S., Eu, K. W., Ooi, L. L. and Wong, W. K. (2006) Perforation of the gastrointestinal tract secondary to ingestion of foreign bodies. *World Journal of Surgery*, **30**(3), 372–7.

Hibberts, F. (2010/2011) Assessing rectal bleeding: a common symptom of haemorrhoids. *Gastrointestinal Nursing*, **8**(10), 16–20.

Howard, T. J., Plaskon, L. A., Wiebke, E. A., Wilcox, M. G. and Madura, J. A. (1996) Nonocclusive mesenteric ischemia remains a diagnostic dilemma. *American Journal of Surgery*, **171**, 405–8.

Iddan, G., Meron, G., Glukhovsky, A. and Swain, P. (2000) Wireless capsule endoscopy, Nature 405:417 May

Lewis, S. J. and Heaton, K. W. (1997) Stool form scale as a useful guide to intestinal transit time. *Scandinavian Journal of Gastroenterology*, **32**(9), 920–4.

Looker, A. C., Dallman, P. R., Carroll, M. D. and Johnson, C. L. (1997) Prevalence of iron deficiency in the United States. *Journal of the American Medical Association*, **277**, 973–6.

Marieb, E. (2003) The digestive system and body metabolism. In: *Essentials of Human Anatomy and Physiology*, 7th edn (ed. E. Marieb), Chapter 14. Benjamin Cummings, London.

Marieb, E. and Hoehn, K. (2007) The digestive system. In: *Human Anatomy and Physiology*, 7th edn (eds. E. Marieb and K. Hoehn), Chapter 23. Pearson Benjamin Cummings, London.

McGrath, A. (2010) Examination of the Abdomen. In: *Physical Assessment for Nurses*, 2nd edn (ed. C. Cox), Chapter 5. Wiley-Blackwell, Oxford.

NDDIC (2007) *Constipation*. National Digestive Diseases Information Clearinghouse, National Institute of Diabetes and Digestive and Kidney Diseases (NIDDK). The NIDDK is part of the National Institutes of Health of the U.S. Department of Health and Human Services.

Netdoctor (2011) *Diarrhoea*. http://www.netdoctor.co.uk/diseases/facts/diarrhoea.htm (accessed 14 December 2011).

Oldenburg, W. A., Lau, L. L., Rodenbery, T. J., Edmonds, H. J. and Burger, C. D. (2004) Acute mesenteric ischemia: a clinical review. *Archives of Internal Medicine*, **164**, 1054–62. (Reprinted by the American Medical Association, downloaded 26 August 2011.)

Prather, C. (2007) Inflammatory and anatomic diseases of the intestine, peritoneum, mesentery, and omentum. In: *Cecil Medicine*, 23rd edn (eds. L. Goldman and D. Ausiello), Chapter 145. Saunders-Elsevier, Philadelphia.

Rockey, D. C. (1999) Occult gastrointestinal bleeding. *New England Journal of Medicine*, **341**, 38–46.

Rockey, D. C. (2005) Occult gastrointestinal bleeding. *Gastroenterology Clinics of North America*, **34**(4), 699–718.

Rockey, D. C. and Cello, J. P. (1993) Evaluation of the gastrointestinal tract in patients with iron-deficiency anaemia. *New England Journal of Medicine*, **329**, 1691–5.

Rockey, D. C., Koch, J., Cello, J. P. and Sanders, L. L. (1998) Relative frequency of upper gastrointestinal and colonic lesions in patients with positive fecal occult-blood tests. *New England Journal of Medicine*, **339**, 153–9.

Rockey, D. C., Auslander, A. and Greenberg, P. D. (1999) Detection of upper gastrointestinal blood with fecal occult blood tests. *American Journal of Gastroenterology*, 94, 344–50.

Russo, M. W., Wei, J. T., Thiny, M. T., Gangarosa, L. M., Brown, A., Ringel, Y., Shaheen, N. J. and Sandler, R. S. (2004) Digestive and liver diseases statistics, 2004. *Gastroenterology*, **126**, 1448–53.

Swartz, M. (2006) The abdomen. In: *Physical Diagnosis, History and Examination*, 5th edn (ed. M. Swartz), Chapter 16. W. B. Saunders, London.

Talley, N. and O'Connor, S. (1998) The abdomen. In *Pocket Clinical Examination* (eds. N. Talley and S. O'Connor), Chapter 4. Blackwell Science, Oxford.

Talley, N. and O'Connor, S. (2006) The gastrointestinal system. In: *Clinical Examination: a Systematic Guide to Physical Diagnosis*, 5th edn (eds. N. Talley and S. O'Connor), Chapter 5. Churchill Livingstone, Edinburgh.

Additional Internet resources

http://www.corecharity.org.uk/Windy-symptoms-Flatulence-belching-bloating-and-break-ing-wind.html (accessed 20 April 2011)

http://digestive.niddk.nih.gov/ddiseases/pubs/pancreatitis/ (accessed 20 April 2011)

http://www.emedicinehealth.com/rectal_pain/page3_em.htm (accessed 20 April 2011)

http://www.medicinenet.com/appendicitis/page2.htm (accessed 25 May 2011)

http://knol.google.com/k/occult-gastrointestinal-bleeding (accessed 25 May 2011)

http://digestive.niddk.nih.gov/ddiseases/pubs/pancreatitis/ (accessed 25 May 2011)

http://www.medicinenet.com/appendicitis/page2.htm (accessed 25 May 2011)

http://www.nlm.nih.gov/medlineplus/ency/article/000212.htm (accessed 25 May 2011)

http://www.corecharity.org.uk/Windy-symptoms-Flatulence-belching-bloating-and-break-ing-wind.html (accessed 28 November 2011)

http://www.cndonurse.com/articles/2007/03/gi-perforations.aspx (accessed 28 November 2011)

CHAPTER 6

Tumours of the gastrointestinal tract

Daniel Apau

Introduction

In this chapter common gastrointestinal (GI) tumours including: tumours of the oesophagus, gastric cancer, gastrointestinal stromal tumours (GISTs), pancreatic cancer, small bowel cancer and colorectal cancer will be considered. Global nursing assessment, care planning and interventions for patients with tumours of the GI tract will be elaborated on.

The digestive tract is a major site of cancer in humans with an unequal distribution of incidents among the component sites, from the oesophagus to the anus (Parkin *et al.*, 2005). GI tumours are associated with more mortalities than any other organ system of the body; although gastric cancer is second to lung cancer in the number of individual tumours of the body (Axon, 2001).

By reading this chapter and carrying out the proposed activities you should achieve the following learning outcomes:

■ Improve your knowledge of tumours of the GI tract
■ Understand the management options available in treating tumours of the GI tract
■ Discuss the nursing care required when managing patients with or recovering from tumours of the GI tract

Cancer of the oesophagus

Cancer of the oesophagus is more predominant in those aged 60–70 years with progressive dysphagia, which is the primary symptom presented initially (Fairclough and Silk, 2009). The two most frequently occurring oesophageal cancers are squamous cell carcinoma (SCC) and adenocarcinoma. SCC accounts for most of the cancers that occur in the upper two thirds of the oesophagus (40% are in the upper third and 15%

in the middle third) and adenocarcinoma accounts for most of the cancers in the lower third of the oesophagus (45%) (Fitzgerald, 2010; Fairclough and Silk , 2009). A columnar-lined metaplasia of the distal oesophagus known as Barrett's oesophagus has been linked to over 80% of all adenocarcinomas of the oesophagus (Fitzgerald, 2010; Lagergren, 2006).

Epidemiology and pathophysiology

An increase in the incidence of adenocarcinoma of the oesophagus over the past 20 to 30 years in the Western world is attributed to changes in diagnostics procedures, tumour classification and general awareness of the disease (Lagergren, 2006). Fitzgerald (2010) however, attributes the increase in incidence to increased oesophageal reflux disease, a rise in obesity and a reduced prevalence of *Helicobacter pylori* (*H. pylori*). Other risk factors include tobacco smoking, high alcohol intake, breast cancer that has been treated with radiotherapy, use of anti-inflammatory drugs and a diet high in total and saturated fats (Fitzgerald, 2010; Pera *et al.*, 2005; Wong and Fitzgerald, 2005).

There are approximately 12,000 new cases of oesophageal cancer per year in the UK predominantly in males with an incidence of SCC of about 5–10 per 100,000 whereas adenocarcinoma accounts for 5.0–8.7 per 100,000 (Fitzgerald, 2010). Oesophageal cancer has a high tendency to metastasise into the surrounding nodes as a result of the absence of serosa and extensive submucosal lymphatic drainage (Taylor, 1986). Metastasis of oesophageal cancer is usually through the longitudinal and circumferential wall with the gastric cardia offering no barrier to the spread through submucosal veins and lymphatics to produce isolated tumours at a distance from the original site (Watson, 1994). In advanced stages, oesophageal cancer can spread into the tracheal bronchial tree, pleura, pericardium, aorta and/ or the vertebrae.

Signs and symptoms

The most common universal presentation of oesophageal cancer is dysphagia (difficulty in swallowing) which can progress from a slight sensation of food hold up to progressive dysphagia of solids and eventually to liquids or the individual unable to swallow anything including saliva. The onset of dysphagia, however, may indicate advanced tumour with possible supraclavicular and cervical lymphadenopathy. Metastasis to the laryngeal nerves can lead to hoarseness of the voice whilst narrowing of the oesophagus can cause odynophagia (painful swallowing in the oropharynx or oesophagus) from distension during swallowing (Watson, 1994). Table 6.1 illustrates some of the symptoms of oesophageal cancer.

Table 6.1 Symptoms commonly associated with oesophageal cancer

Frequent	Infrequent
Progressive dysphagia	Hoarseness of voice
Weight loss	Oesophageal pleural fistula
Chronic iron deficiency anaemia	
Pain on swallowing	
Chronic cough	
Coughing up (expectorating) blood	

Endoscopy remains the diagnostic tool providing histological and cytological proof of carcinoma in about 90% of all cases through biopsy and endoscopic brushings (Shields, 2004). Barium swallow has been useful in differentiating dysphagia from other motility disorders. Imaging such as CT and MRI scans are beneficial in exploring and detecting metastasis (refer to Chapter 9 for further information on radiological studies). Staging of oesophageal cancer using the TNM (tumour, node, metastasis) system (see Table 6.2) is essential to determine optimal management through radical therapy for all patients.

Table 6.2 TNM system used in staging oesophageal cancer (adapted from UICC, 2009).

Primary tumour (T)	
TX	Primary tumour cannot be evaluated
T0	No evidence of primary tumour
Tis	Carcinoma *in situ* (CIS; abnormal cells are present but have not spread to neighbouring tissues; although not cancer, CIS may become cancer and is sometimes called pre-invasive cancer)
T1, T2, T3, T4	Size and/or extent of the primary tumour

Regional lymph nodes (N)	
NX	Regional lymph nodes cannot be evaluated
N0	No regional lymph node involvement
N1, N2, N3	Involvement of regional lymph nodes (number of lymph nodes and/or extent of spread)

Distant metastasis (M)	
MX	Distant metastasis cannot be evaluated
M0	No distant metastasis
M1	Distant metastasis is present

The TNM system is based on the extent of the tumour (T), the extent of spread to the lymph nodes (N), and the presence of distant metastasis (M). A number is added to each letter to indicate the size or extent of the primary tumour and the extent of cancer spread.

Management

Survival rates associated with oesophageal cancer are poor, with five-year survival rates of stages 1, 2, 3 and 4 of about 80%, 30%, 18% and 4% respectively (Fairclough and Silk, 2010). Surgery provides the best chance of cure. Surgical resection must be considered in relatively fit patients with favourable tumours of the middle and lower third of the oesophagus (Watson, 1994). Other treatment options include Endoscopic Mucosal Resection (EMR), laser treatment and stenting, chemotherapy and radiotherapy.

> **Activity**
> Consider the type of psychological support a patient might need after being given a diagnosis of oesophageal cancer. Giving a patient a diagnosis like cancer or telling patients that they have a poor prognosis is termed 'breaking bad news'.

Gastric tumours

Gastric tumours are either epithelial or stromal in origin with malignant adenocarcinomas being the most common finding. Benign gastric adenomas and GI stromal tumours (GISTs) are less common and usually discovered during routine gastroscopy or acute GI haemorrhage (Patel and Allum, 2011).

Benign gastric tumours (BGTs)

Benign gastric tumours, although rare, are often found incidentally during routine investigations and can range from solid tumours to gastric mucosal inflammation. BGTs do not produce common clinical problems but are reported in about 5–25% of autopsies, with polyps accounting for about 3.1% (Park and Lauwers, 2007).

Epidemiology and pathophysiology

BGTs have unknown aetiology; but there is a strong relationship between type A atrophic gastritis and inflammatory polyps. They occur equally in men and women with a median age of between 50 and 70 years (Muller *et al.*, 1987). BGTs cover a wide range of pathologies, ranging from solid tumours to inflammatory lesions with difficult differentiation from pre-malignant lesions. BGTs are usually made up of regenerative hyperplastic polyps and benign adenomatous gastric polyps. Other BGT lesions are mesenchymal tumours which arise from any of the connective tissues of the stomach. Leiomyoblastomas arise from the longitudinal and circular muscle coats of the stomach and gastric lipomas originate from the mucosa of the antrum extending into the gastric lumen; sometimes inducing necrosis and haemorrhage (Miettinen and Lasota, 2001).

Management
BGTs are associated with uncommon clinical symptoms hence management depends on histology. Endoscopy of lesions and regular gastroscopic support are the main management plans.

Activity
Read Chapter 9 and initiate a plan for how you will prepare a patient for an endoscopic examination.

Gastric cancer
Gastric cancer is the fourth most common cancer in the world with incidence peaking with age between 50 to 70 years (Fairclough and Silk, 2010). In the UK, gastric cancer is the eighth most common cancer in males and the thirteenth in females, with about 7,784 new cases being diagnosed in 2007 (Cancer Research UK, 2011a). Survival rates are about 42% at 12 months and 24% at 5 years from date of diagnosis (Berrino, 2003; Cancer Research UK, 2011a).

Epidemiology and pathophysiology
H. pylori has been aetiologically linked to gastric cancer, and the simultaneous decline of gastric cancer along with decline in *H. pylori* infections strongly supports the link (Moayyedi *et al.*, 2002). There is growing evidence that diet plays an important role in a predisposition to gastric cancer. Diets high in salt, high meat intake and processed meat have been associated with an increased risk of gastric cancer, whilst non-starchy vegetables, low salt diet and vegetarian meals protect against gastric cancer (Cancer Research UK, 2011a; Fairclough and Silk, 2010). In addition to the above risk factors, other causes of gastric cancer have been attributed to medications such as the use of aspirin, medical conditions

such as gastro-oesophageal reflux disease, body weight, lack of physical activity, radiation, and occupational and environmental exposures to dust and pollen (Cancer Research UK, 2011a).

First-degree relatives of gastric cancer patients have a relatively higher risk of developing gastric cancer from possible environmental causes than a genetic or hereditary predisposition as previously thought (Fairclough and Silk, 2010). Patients who suffer with pernicious anaemia are at risk of developing gastric cancer due to atrophic gastritis which can ensue with chronic pernicious anaemia (Berrino, 2003).

Most malignant tumours of the stomach are epithelial in origin; therefore adenocarcinoma constitutes about 95% of all cases (Bridgewater and Pereira, 2010). Adenocarcinoma of the interstitial type is usually found in old age and has a good survival rate. Interstitial adenocarcinoma is associated with atrophic gastritis, whilst diffuse adenocarcinomas tend to infiltrate the gastric wall and may spread to other parts of the stomach (Fairclough and Silk, 2010). Inflammation induced by *H. pylori* infection is believed to activate the nuclear factor kappa-light-chain-enhancer of activated B cells (NF-kB) with pro-inflammatory mediators which lead to targeting of gastric cells and promotion of tumour growth factor by inhibiting apoptosis. The process results in atrophic gastritis with loss of glandular tissues and subsequent development of metaplasia, dysplasia and the onset of gastric cancer (Cancer Research UK, 2011a; Lee and Feldman, 2006).

Signs and symptoms

Symptoms of gastric cancer do not appear until late in the disease process. About half of all gastric cancer cases are discovered at screening with no symptoms and less than 2% of patients presenting to their GPs with dyspepsia symptoms for the first time go on to develop gastric cancer (Fairclough and Silk, 2010; Cancer Research UK, 2011a). Due to the vagueness of initial symptoms, and difficulty differentiating between benign tumours and malignancy, national guidelines are in place to help practitioners identify which patients need referral to a specialist in the UK (NICE, 2011). Weight loss, epigastric pain, indigestion, loss of appetite and tiredness are often some of the presenting symptoms, with about 50% having a palpable epigastric mass and supraclavicular lymphadenopathy (Fairclough and Silk, 2010).

Diagnosis and management

Diagnosis of gastric cancer is made following gastroscopy and histological analysis of biopsies or washings. A negative biopsy does not usually rule out carcinoma and continuous assessment should be carried out for all suspicious lesions during gastroscopy. Other investigations, such as barium meal, CT scan, endoscopic scan, trans-abdominal ultrasound, positron emission tomography (PET) and CT/PET, can help delineate carcinoma *in situ*.

There is limited medical treatment for gastric cancer and surgical removal of the lesions remains the most effective form for patients who are fit for surgical operation. Non-ulcerated or infiltrated lesions can be endoscopically removed. Chemotherapy and radiation are sometimes used in conjunction with surgery.

Activity
Review the clinical guidelines for the administration of chemotherapy in the setting in which you are training or work.

Gastrointestinal stromal tumours (GISTs)

GISTs are uncommon types of neoplasm which can occur anywhere along the GI tract. GISTs are classified as sarcomas, as their formation begin in the connective tissue such as fat, muscle, blood vessels, deep skin tissues, nerves, cartilages and synovial tissues (Cancer Research UK, 2011b). About 60–70% of GISTs arise in the stomach with 20–30% originating in the small intestine and about 10% originating in the oesophagus, colon, and rectum (Miettinen and Lasota, 2001). Most GISTs in the GI tract originate in the stromal cells which align the tract to aid peristalsis, but they can also occur in extra intestinal sites of the abdomen or pelvis, such as the omentum, mesentery and retroperitoneum (Demetri, 2006).

Epidemiology and pathophysiology
GISTs are the most common mesenchymal neoplasm of the GI tract and third in the prevalence of all GI neoplasms (Demetri, 2006). There are about 200–900 new cases of GISTs in the UK per annum and these occur mainly in the 50 to 70 years age group (Cancer Research UK, 2011b; Fairclough and Silk, 2010). GISTs are submucosal lesions which can range in size from 1 cm to 40 cm diameter with size and tumour characteristics such as mitotic rate determining long-term survival (Corless *et al.*, 2004).

Signs and symptoms
GI bleed is the most common clinical manifestation with about 40–60% of patients presenting with haematemesis or melaena usually due to ulceration of

lesions (Blanke *et al.*, 2005). Patients may also complain of early satiety, feelings of abdominal fullness and vague non-specific abdominal pain (Corless *et al.*, 2004). Physical examination may yield a palpable abdominal mass but rarely demonstrates any valuable findings.

Pancreatic cancer

Pancreatic cancer has one of the lowest incidences of neoplasms but a high mortality rate, approaching almost 100% at 5 years post-diagnosis (Lowenfels and Maisonneuve, 2006).

Epidemiology and pathophysiology

Pancreatic cancer ranks as thirteenth in incidence but eighth in mortality (Anderson *et al.*, 2006; Lowenfels and Maisonneuve, 2006). The incidence of pancreatic cancer is rare under the age of 45 years and affects more males than females with a higher incidence in black males in the USA (American Cancer Society, 2011). In the UK the incidence is about 12.4/100,000 population per year, with about 7,684 cases of pancreatic cancers reported. The distribution among males and females remains the same although it is higher in males for age standardised mortality rates (Office for National Statistics, 2010; Lombard and Gillmore, 2010). About 95% of pancreatic malignancies originate from the ductal and acinar cells with features of adenocarcinoma and the islet cells accounting for about 1–2% (Castillo and Jimenez, 2006). Ductal adenocarcinoma incidence is about 85–90% of all pancreatic tumours.

Tumours of the head of the pancreas tend to obstruct the distal common bile and pancreatic ducts leading to jaundice. Metastasis from the pancreatic cancer initially involves the regional lymph nodes, the liver, surrounding visceral organs and less often the lungs (Solcia *et al.*, 1997). Pancreatic cancer is multi-focal in aetiology, but strong links have been established with smoking, diabetes, chronic pancreatitis, genetics and alcohol consumption.

Cigarette smoking has been shown to contribute to about 25% of all pancreatic cancer cases, with smokers tending to develop the condition 10 years earlier than non-smokers (Lombard and Gilmore, 2010). Strong correlation exists between diabetes mellitus and pancreatic cancer, with a considerable number of pancreatic cancer patients diagnosed with type 2 diabetes two years before developing cancer (Stevens *et al.*, 2007). Up to about 10% of all pancreatic cancer patients may have a genetic cause from possible susceptibility to organic compounds in the environment (Lombard and Gilmore, 2010).

Clinical features

Presentations and features might differ depending on whether the cancer developed in the head, body or tail of the pancreas, but typical clinical features include weight loss, abdominal or epigastric pain and jaundice. Pain features in about 50–80% of all patient presentations. The pain is usually described as dull and vague and is frequently exacerbated by ingestion of food, possibly due to pancreatic stimulation to produce digestive enzymes (Russell, 1994).

Weight loss, which can be rapid and progressive, occurs in about 90% of all patients due to possible malabsorption caused by blockade of the pancreatic duct. Cholestatic jaundice is usually the first symptom in about 10–30% of all patients and results from either obstruction of the common bile duct or possible hepatic metastasis. Patients with jaundice may also experience pruritus, steatorrhoea and passing of dark brown urine (Russell, 1994).

Activity

Patients experiencing pain from pancreatic tumours generally do not like to eat, as eating increases their pain. Weight loss is a serious problem in this patient population. List the interventions you think should be administered by the nurse so that patients are able to eat more comfortably.

Tumours of the small intestine

Small bowel tumours may be benign polyps, lipomas or malignant and generally affect persons in the fifth, sixth and seventh decades of life, with equal distribution among both sexes (Calam and Williamson, 1994). Small bowel neoplasms are rare due to relative resistance and account for 3–6% of all GI tumours and about 0.2–0.3% of all malignancies (Bridgewater and Pereira, 2010; Fairclough and Silk, 2010). The rarity of small bowel neoplasms has been attributed to increased transit time of bowel content and inaccessibility of the small intestine for investigations; hence most neoplasms are found during routine laparotomy and at autopsy (Calam and Williamson, 1994).

Epidemiology and pathophysiology

In the UK about 1000 people are diagnosed every year with small bowel cancer (Cancer Research UK, 2011c). About 40% of all small bowel cancers are adenocarcinomas involving the epithelial cells of the GI tract and mainly found in the duodenum whilst carcinoid tumours account for about 30% and mainly affect the appendix or the ileum (Cancer Research UK, 2011c). Small bowel adenocarcinomas tend to conglomerate away from the colon and toward the gastric end of the small intestine, with approximately 50% arising in the duodenum, 30% in the jejunum and 20% in the ileum (Lowenfels and Sonni, 1997). Primary carcinomas of the small intestine usually arise in the duodenum whilst secondary carcinomas are likely to have metastasised from the breast or pulmonary cavity (Callam and Williamson, 1994).

Signs and symptoms

Symptoms of a small bowel neoplasm depend on the location of the lesion, size and staging. Most patients are usually asymptomatic, but about 90% develop symptoms which correlate to the type, location and characteristics of the neoplasm (Cancer Research UK, 2011c). Symptoms can include non-specific, dull epigastric pain (especially if close to the duodenum), changes in bowel habits and consistency, weight loss, anaemia, nausea and vomiting and bowel obstruction (Cancer Research UK, 2011c).

Management

Management of small bowel neoplasm depends on the lesion, location, size and histological characteristics. Generally surgery, chemotherapy and radiotherapy are the main interventions.

Activity

Review the pre-operative preparation that nurses provide to patients that are scheduled for bowel surgery.

Colorectal cancer

Colorectal cancer is the third most common form of malignancy; especially in the developed world, with a high morbidity rate as one of the attributes worldwide. In the UK there are about 110 new cases diagnosed each day. It is the most common malignancy after breast cancer in women, and in men it rates third after prostate and lung cancer (Cancer Research UK, 2011d).

Epidemiology and pathophysiology

Available information indicates there were about 34,889 newly registered cases of colorectal cancer in the UK in 2002, and about 16,259 deaths from colorectal cancer in 2008 with the highest occurrence of deaths in people aged over 65 years (Cancer Research UK, 2011d). About two-thirds of all colorectal tumours occur in the colon and one third in the rectum with the left side of the colon from the splenic flexure registering about 60% of all tumours (Cancer Research UK, 2011d). About 90% of all colorectal cancers are adenocarcinomas which originate from benign polyps that commonly develop from the colonic mucosa (Midgley and Kerr, 1999). Progression of benign adenomatous polyps to invasive adenocarcinoma involves genetic mutation of the adenomatous polyposis gene to familial adenomatous polyposis which is a rare hereditary syndrome (Vogelstein *et al.*, 1988). A small percentage of colorectal cancers are linked to a strong genetic predisposition with over 75% of all cases arising in people over 65 years of age (Bridgewater and Pereira, 2010).

Risk factors

Diet plays an important factor in colorectal cancers with an increased incidence in populations with a diet rich in red meat and processed meat. There is an increase in incidence in migrants or populations who have adopted 'Western diets' rich in meat and processed meats (Cancer Research UK, 2011d). A diet poor in fibre, high in fat, a lack of fruits and vegetables, deficient in folate, calcium and vitamins B and D increases the risk of colorectal cancer (Cancer Research UK, 2011d).

Obesity increases the risk of bowel cancer by 25% in women and about 50% in men, with a significant risk reduction in women with a Body Mass Index (BMI) of less than 25 (Moghaddam *et al.*, 2007). Furthermore a sedentary lifestyle without high levels of physical activity increases the risk of colorectal cancer by about 13–14% (Wolin *et al.*, 2011).

Some pharmacological agents have been shown to reduce the risk of incidence of colorectal cancer such as consumption of low dose aspirin daily, Hormone Replacement Therapy (HRT) and the oral contraceptive pill (Cancer Research UK, 2011d). The risk of developing colorectal cancer rises sharply after age 40 years, with 90% of all cases occurring in persons over 50 years of age (Cancer Research UK, 2011b).

Signs and symptoms

As with all neoplasms of the GI tract, the signs and symptoms presented will depend on the location, size, stage and histological characteristics of the lesion. Distal lesions are likely to produce obstruction and bleeding with stools which may affect bowel habits and feelings of inadequate emptying with possible constipation. Persons with asymptomatic cancers often have occult blood loss with bleeding rates increasing with increasing size of the lesion (Bresalier, 2006).

Due to the narrow lumen size of the proximal colon, lesions in the descending and sigmoid colon may cause obstruction and the patient might complain of colicky type pain as well as having bouts of constipation (Bresalier, 2006). In general weight loss, anaemia due to occult blood and bowel obstruction may be present in patients.

Management

Management of colorectal cancer depends on the size and location of the lesion, condition of patient, stage and histological characteristics of the tumour. Surgery, chemotherapy, radiotherapy and palliation are the current therapeutic interventions available.

Activity

The National Health Service (NHS) in England has established a Bowel Cancer Screening Programme. This programme is aimed toward detecting bowel cancer early in its development when successful treatment and cure is more likely. Screening is offered to people aged 60–69 who are registered with a GP in England. Review the procedure for screening that has been developed. (Note that many patients do not take up the screening programme because they find it repulsive.) Identify how you can help patients comply with the screening test procedure.

Post-diagnosis assessment, pre- and post-therapeutic interventions for patients with a GI tumour

In this section, post-diagnosis assessment and care pre- and post-therapeutic interventions will be described in relation to a patient with a GI tumour. Nursing assessment, diagnosis, care planning and interventions for patients with GI tumours are directed towards preparation of patients and relatives for surgery, radiotherapy, chemotherapy and provision of palliative care. It is imperative that comprehensive assessment of the GI system is undertaken including history and physical assessment to extrapolate rich data capable of aiding diagnosis.

Subjective data

History taking

History taking should seek to extrapolate from the patient any symptoms suggestive of neoplasm. A complete history should elicit any abdominal pain, dyspepsia, diarrhoea, changes in bowel habits and consistency of stools, jaundice, nausea and vomiting and change in appetite. Table 6.3 illustrates some of the factors to consider during history taking and when assessing for pain in possible GI neoplasm. History taking should be holistic to cover all aspects of the patient's cultural and religious beliefs.

Table 6.3 Factors to consider during history taking and when assessing for pain.

Associated symptoms	Weight loss; may indicate malabsorption caused by neoplasm Anaemia: may indicate bleeding from the GI tract or vitamin B_{12} synthesis in the GI tract Nausea and vomiting may indicate reduced peristalsis from possible obstruction Changes in stools consistency: steatorrhoea may indicate liver or pancreatic problems Early satiety may indicate the presence of lesion in the stomach
History of pain	Rapidity of onset, progression and sustainability is a measure of the severity of the underlying disorder
Progression of pain	Progression of pain is an important factor as pain from a neoplasm will progress in line with increasing size of the lesion
Location of pain	Location of pain will indicate which part of the GI system is affected. Pain in the epigastric region is likely to involve the oesophagus, stomach or duodenum. Changes in location of pain could indicate progression from visceral to parietal irritation which can be an indication of progressing severity of the patient's condition
Aggravating and alleviating factors	Pain characteristics that change with different activities is significant. Patients complaining of pain following food ingestion are significant, as this could be due to be neoplastic irritation from the food, or forceful expansion from tumour-induced obstruction or in the case of pancreatic tumour
Past medical history	Some medical conditions increase risks of neoplasm of the GI tract such as chronic pancreatitis, Crohn's disease, coeliac disease
Medication	To assess medication risks such as use of NSAIDs
Family history	To elicit genetic and hereditary predisposition
Social history	To rule out a possible environmental cause of a neoplasm

Objective data

Physical assessment

Physical assessment should use the art of inspection, auscultation, percussion, palpation and other manoeuvres to elicit information to aid diagnosis.

Inspection

Inspection should not be restricted to the abdomen but rather the entire body, from head to toes. The appearance of the patient should be observed for signs of malnutrition. The lips and oral cavity should be inspected for inflammation, lesions and odour, as many disorders, including cancer, may manifest in changes in the oral cavity such as stomatitis, leukoplakia and hairy tongue. The sclera and conjunctiva of the eyes should be inspected for the presence of jaundice or anaemia. The abdomen should be inspected for distension, ascites, striae, caput medusae and/ or spider naevi, which could indicate liver neoplasm. Finally, the rectal and perianal area should be inspected for any lesions suggestive of neoplasm.

Palpation

Palpation enables assessment of local and generalised tenderness as well as identifying landmarks and masses. Deep palpation will elicit borders of organs and solid masses. Palpation is vital in eliciting colorectal cancer. A rectal examination should be performed by qualified personnel in all cases of rectal pain and a history suspicious of colon or rectal neoplasm.

Percussion

Percussion is required to determine whether underlying tissues or organs are air-filled, fluid-filled or solid. This is undertaken by using the tip of the right middle finger (the plexor finger) to strike the distal interphalangeal joint of the pleximeter finger. Percussion is needed to determine the borders of organs and any to reveal peritoneal irritation in abdominal pain. Any large areas of dullness may indicate the presence of abdominal mass or tumour.

Auscultation

Auscultation, which is the act of listening for sounds using a stethoscope, should be done with the patient positioned comfortably in the supine position if possible. Auscultation of the abdomen should start from the right upper quadrant in a clockwise manner, noting bowel sounds and characteristics suggestive of gastrointestinal obstruction.

Nursing diagnosis

Based on assessment of the patient with a GI tumour, nursing diagnoses may include the following:

- Nausea and vomiting caused by GI stasis or other therapeutic interventions
- Anxiety relating to diagnosis of tumour and impending therapeutic interventions
- Pain related to the presence of a tumour and its effect on surrounding tissues
- Imbalanced nutritional and fluid volume deficit from dysphagia, GI obstruction and decreased volume intake
- Impaired skin integrity
- Impaired body image

Some of the potential problems following therapeutic interventions may include:

- Intraperitoneal/systemic infection
- Risk of haemorrhage/haemodynamic instability
- Damping syndrome
- Risk of aspiration

Care planning and nursing interventions

The major goals for the patient following diagnosis of GI tumour include relieving anxiety, relieving pain, establishing optimal nutrition, education about the patient's condition and adjustment to body image and lifestyle changes. The nature of nursing interventions and care planning for patients with GI tumours will depend on the presenting condition and outlined therapeutic intervention of the patient.

Reducing anxiety

A diagnosis of any form of tumour can impose considerable psychological challenges to the patient and the family. An important part of care for the patient with a diagnosis of GI tumour is to allay all fears and anxieties that the patient and relatives might have regarding the condition. The patient needs encouragement to express and ask questions about any fears they might have. Adequate psychological preparation for therapeutic procedures and post-procedures is vital to ensure optimal treatment. The patient should be directed to any available support for the type of condition they have.

Relieving pain

The nursing intervention for relieving pain will depend on the nature of neoplasm and therapeutic intervention advocated or performed. Post-operative pain, therapeutic intervention-induced pain, and pain from a lesion or lesions and surrounding tissues is relieved by assessing the patient's pain using a pain scoring chart and administering prescribed analgesia accordingly. Pain experienced by patients should not be underestimated. Therefore a concern regarding addiction to analgesia should not feature in the medical and surgical regimen prescribed for the patient.

Promoting adequate hydration and nutritional intake

Most patients at time of diagnosis will have a degree of anaemia and dehydration. Nutritional assessment is vital to provide the high protein and caloric intake required either enterally or parenterally prior to any therapeutic interventions. Patients with total or partial gastrectomies will lack intrinsic factor and should have their vitamin B_{12} monitored and replaced accordingly. The patient's weight and height should be obtained on admission and weekly weights instigated to monitor for changes during care. Fluid balance should be monitored and adequate replacement effected.

Impaired skin integrity

Skin integrity might be compromised post-surgery, post-chemotherapy or by other therapeutic interventions that have the ability to interfere with cellular integrity. If the patient is bed-bound pressure area care should be instigated after assessing risks using tools like the Braden scale or Waterlow scale. The use of emollients and loose clothing should be encouraged to avoid friction and shearing of skin.

Disturbed body image

Almost invariably, therapeutic interventions for GI tumours will have a considerable impact on the body image of the patient. The use of chemotherapy or radiation might alter body image by causing alopecia and/or decreased sexual function for example. It is vital that patients are assessed for potential challenges to their self esteem. Collaborative approaches involving other specialists in managing the patient's challenges are essential in meeting the patient's needs.

Nausea and vomiting

Patients might experience nausea and vomiting from therapeutic interventions such as chemotherapy, radiotherapy and gut stasis from obstruction. It is important that the patient is assessed for risk of aspiration, and appropriate action such as passing of a nasogastric tube implemented. The patient should be given required antiemetics and good oral hygiene should be provided.

> **Activity**
> Prioritise the care that a patient, post-surgery for a GI tumour, should receive.

Summary

This chapter has considered GI tumours, including tumours of the oesophagus, gastric cancer, gastrointestinal stromal tumours (GISTs), pancreatic cancer, small bowel cancer and colorectal cancer. Global nursing assessment, care planning and interventions for patients with tumours of the GI tract were elaborated. It has been noted that GI tumours are associated with more mortalities than any other organ system of the body, with gastric cancer second to lung cancer for individual tumours of the body. Nursing management plans that reduce anxiety, relieve pain, promote adequate hydration and nutritional intake, maintain skin integrity, provide collaborative support in instances where the patient is experiencing a disturbed body image and effectively control nausea and vomiting are the foundation for the provision of good patient care.

References

American Cancer Society (2011) *Cancer Facts and Figures for African Americans 2009–2010* [Online]. Available at: http://www.cancer.org/acs/groups/content/@nho/documents/document/cffaa20092010pdf.pdf (accessed June 2011).

Anderson, K. E., Mark, T., Silverman, D. (2006) Cancer of the pancreas. In: *Cancer Epidemiology and Prevention*, 3rd edn (eds. D. Schottenfeld and J. F. Fraumeni Jr). Oxford University Press, New York.

Axon, A. T. R. (2001) Preface. In: *Clinical Gastroenterology: PreMalignant Conditions of the GI Tract: Possibilities for Prevention.* Baillière Tindall, London.

Berrino, F. (2003) The EUROCARE study: strength, limitation and perspectives of population based comparative survival studies. *Annals of Oncology*, **14**(5), v9–v13.

Blanke, C., Eisenberg, B. L. and Heinrich, M. C. (2005) Epidemiology of GISTs. *American Journal of Gastroenterology*, **100**(10), 2366.

Bresalier, R. S. (2006) Malignant neoplasm of the large intestine. In: *Sleisenger and Fordtran's GI and Liver Disease*, 8th edn (eds. M. Feldman, L. S. Friedman and L. J. Brandt). Saunders Elsevier, Philadelphia.

Bridgewater, J. A. and Pereira, S. P. (2010) Cancers of the GI tract. In: *Oxford Textbook of Medicine*, 5th edn (eds. D. A. Warrell, T. M. Cox and J. D. Firth). Oxford University Press, Oxford.

Calam, J. and Williamson, R. C. N. (1994) Neoplastic and miscellaneous diseases of the small intestine. In: *Diseases of the Gut and Pancreas*, 2nd edn (eds. J. J. Misiewicz, R. E. Pounder and C. W. Venables). Blackwell Scientific Publications, London.

Cancer Research UK (2011a) *Stomach Cancer Incidence* [Online]. Available at: http://info.cancerresearchuk.org/cancerstats/types/stomach/incidence/ (accessed June 2011).

Cancer Research UK (2011b). *What is Gastrointestinal Stromal Tumour?* [Online]. Available at: http://www.cancerhelp.org.uk/about-cancer/cancer-questions/what-is-the-treatment-for-gist-gastrointestinal-stromal-tumour (accessed June 2011).

Cancer Research UK (2011c) *Small Bowel Cancer Question* [Online]. Available at: http://www.cancerhelp.org.uk/about-cancer/cancer-questions/small-bowel-cancer-question (accessed June 2011).

Cancer Research UK (2011d) *Bowel (Colorectal) Cancer. UK Incidence Statistics* [Online]. Available at: http://info.cancerresearchuk.org/cancerstats/types/bowel/incidence/ (accessed June 2011).

Castillo, C. F. and Jimenez, R. E. (2006) Pancreatic cancer, cystic pancreatic neoplasm and other non endocrine pancreatic tumours. In: *Sleisenger and Fordtran's GI and Liver Disease*, 8th edn (eds. M. Feldman, L. S. Friedman and L. J. Brandt). Saunders Elsevier, Philadelphia.

Corless, C. L., Fletcher, J. A. and Heinriech, M. C. (2004) Biology of GI stromal tumours. *Journal of Clinical Oncology*, **22**, 38813–25.

Demetri, G. D. I. (2006) GI stromal tumours. In: *Sleisenger and Fordtran's GI and Liver Disease*, 8th edn (eds. M. Feldman, L. S. Friedman and L. J. Brandt). Saunders Elsevier, Philadelphia.

Fairclough, P. D. and Silk, D. B. A. (2009) GI disease. In: *Kumar and Clark's Clinical Medicine* (eds. P. J. Kumar and M. Clark). Saunders Elsevier, London.

Fitzgerald, R. (2010) Diseases of the oesophagus. In: *Oxford Textbook of Medicine*, 5th edn (eds. D. A. Warrell, T. M. Cox and J. D. Firth). Oxford University Press, Oxford.

Lagergren, J. (2006) Aetiology and risk factors for oesophageal adenocarcinoma: possibilities for chemoprophylaxis. In: *Clinical Gastroenterology: Oesophageal Adenocarcinoma* (ed. G. N. J. Tytgart). Elsevier, Oxford.

Lee, E. L. and Feldman, M. (2006) Gastritis and other gastropathies. In: *Sleisenger and Fordtran's GI and Liver Disease*, 8th edn (eds. M. Feldman, L. S. Friedman and L. J. Brandt). Saunders Elsevier, Philadelphia.

Lombard, M. and Gilmore, I. (2010) Tumours of the pancreas. In: *Oxford Textbook of Medicine*, 5th edn (eds. D. A. Warrell, T. M. Cox and J. D. Firth). Oxford University Press, Oxford.

Lowenfels, A. B. and Sonni, A. (1977) Distribution of small bowel tumours. *Cancer Letters*, **3**(1–2), 83–6.

Lowenfels, A. B. and Maisonneuve, P. (2006) Epidemiology of and risk factors for pancreatic cancer. In: *Clinical Gastroenterology: Pancreatic Cancer* (ed. G. N. J. Tytgart). Elsevier, Oxford.

Midgley, R. and Kerr, D. (1999) Colorectal cancer. *Lancet*, **353**, 391–9.

Miettinen, M. and Lasota, J. (2001) GI stromal tumours - definition, clinical histological, immunohistochemical and molecular genetic features and differential diagnosis. *Virchows Archives*, **438**(1), 1–12.

Moayyedi, P., Axon, A., Feltbower, R., Duffett, S., Crocombe, W., Braunholtz, D., Richards, G., Dowell, A. and Forman, D. (2002) Relation of adult lifestyle and socioeconomic factors to the prevalence of *Helicobacter pylori* infection. *International Journal of Epidemiology*, **31**(3), 624–31.

Moghaddam, A. A., Woodward, M. and Huxley, R. (2007) Obesity and risk of colorectal cancer: a meta-analysis of 31 studies with 70,000 events. *Cancer Epidemiology Biomarkers Preview*, 16(12), 2533–47.

Muller, J., Kirchner, T. and Muller-Hermelink, H. K. (1987) Gastric endocrine cell hyperplasia and carcinoid tumours in atropic gastritis type A. *American Journal of Surgical Pathology*, **11**(18), 909–17.

National Institute for Clinical Excellence (NICE) (2011) *Clinical Guideline 27: Referral for Suspected Cancer*. Available at: http://guidance.nice.org.uk/CG27/QuickRefGuide/pdf/English (accessed June 2011).

Office for National Statistics (2010) *Cancer Statistics Registrations: Registrations of Cancer Diagnosed in 2007, England*. HMSO, London.

Parkin, D. M., Whelan, S. L., Ferlay, J., and Storm, H. (2005) *Cancer Incidence in Five Continents*, Vols. I–VIII. International Agency for Research in Cancer, Lyon.

Park, D. Y, and Lauwers, G. Y. (2007) Gastric polyps: classification and management. *Archives of Pathology and Laboratory Medicine*, **132**(4), 633–40.

Patel, H. and Allum, W. H. (2011) Gastric tumours. *Medicine*, **39**(3), 169–72.

Pera, M., Manterola, C., Vidal, O. and Grande, L. (2005) Epidemiology of oesophageal adenocarcinoma. *Journal of Surgical Oncology*, **92**, 151–9.

Russell, R. C. G. (1994) Carcinoma of the pancreas and ampulla of Vater. In: *Diseases of the Gut and Pancreas*, 2nd edn (eds. J. J. Misiewicz, R. E. Pounder and C. W. Venables). Blackwell Scientific Publications, London.

Shields, S. (2004) Malignant esophagus. In: *Gastrointestinal Endoscopy* (eds. J. Dam and R. C. K. Wong). Landes Bioscience, Texas.

Solcia, E., Capella, C. and Kloppel, G. (1997) Tumours of the exocrine pancreas. In: *Tumours of the Pancreas* (eds. E. Solcia, C. Capella and G. Kloppel). Armed Forces Institute of Pathology, Washington DC.

Stevens, R. J., Roddam, A. W. and Beral, V. (2007) Pancreatic cancer in type 1 and young onset diabetes: systematic review and meta-analysis. *British Journal of Cancer*, **96**(3), 507–9.

Taylor, C. R. (1986) Carcinoma of the oesophagus: current imaging options. *American Journal of Gastroenterology*, **81**, 1013–20.

UICC (2009) *Oesophagus*, 7th edn. Union for International Cancer Control [Online]. Available at: http://www.uicc.org/sites/clonesource.agenceinovae.com/files/TNM%20Classification%20of%20Malignant%20Tumours_Website_16%20November%202010_0.pdf (accessed June 2011).

Vogelstein, B., Fearon, E. R., Hamilton, S. R., Kern, S. E., Preisinger, A. C., Leppert, M., Nakamura, Y., White, R., Smits, A. M., and Bos, J. L. (1988) Genetic alterations during colorectal-tumour development. *New England Journal of Medicine*, **319**(9), 525–32.

Watson, A. (1994) Carcinoma of the oesophagus. In: *Diseases of the Gut and Pancreas*, 2nd edn (eds. J. J. Misiewicz, R. E. Pounder and C. W. Venables). Blackwell Scientific Publications, London.

Wolin, K. Y., Yan, Y., and Colditz, G. A. (2011) Physical activity and risk of colon adenoma: a meta-analysis. *British Journal of Cancer*, **104**(5), 882–5.

Wong, A. and Fitzgerald, R. C. (2005) Epidemiologic risk factors for Barrett's oesophagus and associated adenocarcinoma. *Clinical Gastroenterology and Hepatology*, **3**, 1–10.

CHAPTER 7

Malabsorption syndromes

Alison Coutts

Introduction

This chapter considers malabsorption syndromes. The function of the gastrointestinal (GI) tract is to digest foods, so that they are reduced to individual nutrients, which are mostly small, simple molecules, and then absorb them. This chapter is concerned with individuals in whom that process functions imperfectly; thus nutrients are either not digested or the resulting nutrients are not absorbed. The effect on individuals can be devastating, as they experience the double effects of alterations within their bowels and the malnutrition resulting from the poor handling of nutrients.

By reading this chapter and carrying out the proposed activities you should achieve the following learning outcomes:

- Improve your knowledge of malabsorption syndromes
- Describe the pathophysiology associated with malabsorption syndromes
- Discuss the nursing care required when managing patients with malabsorption syndromes

Definition

Malabsorption is not a diagnosis but a range of syndromes that occur when nutrients are not absorbed from within the GI tract. The syndromes vary in their extent and severity, as shown here:

- Selective malabsorption occurs when just one or a very few nutrients fail to be absorbed, but the remainder are absorbed just as they are in a healthy individual.
- Partial malabsorption occurs when all or most nutrients are absorbed unsatisfactorily, although often one or two nutrients are particularly obvious in their absence, such as iron.

- Total malabsorption occurs when there is almost no absorption of any nutrients from the GI tract.

Pathophysiology

The causes of malabsorption are varied, but can be classified into just a few groups:

- Abnormal epithelium, usually due to inflammation or infection
- Structural abnormalities of the GI tract, resulting in reduction in absorptive surface
- Insufficient digestive agents such as insufficiency of pancreatic hormones and failure to absorb bile salts (this is sometimes termed digestive failure)
- Impaired transport

These cannot all be explored in full, but some of the more significant pathologies can be discussed before going on to review caring for patients.

Inflammation and infection

A major cause of malabsorption is inflammatory bowel disease (IBD). IBD is addressed in Chapter 8.

Whipple's disease is a rare systemic infection that particularly infects the GI system. The causative organism is *Tropheryma whipplei*, a bacterium named after George Hoyt Whipple, who first described the disease on 1907. However, at the time Whipple could not isolate the organism. Infection with *T. whipplei* causes the villi of the gut to become thickened so that the mucosa is rendered unable to absorb nutrients. Anyone can develop this infection, although it is more common amongst middle-aged Caucasian men: it is possible that those who develop it have an inability to mount an effective immune response; possibly due to a genetic weakness. Because it is a rare disease it is often difficult to diagnose. A definitive diagnosis requires DNA analysis of the bacterium. This infection requires over a year's treatment with one or more antibiotics. Taken properly the disease can be completely eradicated. Left untreated it is usually fatal.

Human immunodeficiency virus (HIV, the causative organism of acquired immune deficiency disease, AIDS) has a severe effect on nutritional status, partly through the adverse effects on metabolism of the Aids Related Complex (ARC), and is thus a systemic effect. However, there is increasing evidence that HIV directly attacks the gut, and that this attack may not be controlled by drugs that are generally thought to be effective against HIV and the resulting AIDS. It appears that HIV is able to survive in the gut despite long-term and generally effective anti-retroviral treatment (Chun *et al.*, 2008). In the gut it disrupts the normal metabolism and absorption of nutrients, and this contributes to the cachexia often seen in people with advanced AIDS. There is evidence in children of HIV causing malabsorption, leading to iron deficiency anaemia (Castaldo *et al.*, 1996) and lipid deficiency (Carroccio *et al.*, 1998). Similar problems have been found in adults (Carbonnel, 1997). It is worth noting that these researchers found that HIV patients with malabsorption often do not have diarrhoea, which is usually associated with malabsorption, so there is a danger that malabsorption may be overlooked.

The normal GI tract is fully colonised by a wide range of bacteria and fungi. These are not only harmless but actually beneficial. They provide some nutrients, particularly vitamin K. Furthermore, since they fully colonise the GI tract, pathogens are unable to adhere to the walls of the GI tract and are often successfully eradicated by the immune system. The bacteria colonising the large bowel are in dynamic equilibrium, whereby the bacteria are replicating and potentially increasing in number, whilst the host (person) immune system is keeping both the numbers and the sites they colonise in check. As well as that, new (and potentially harmful) bacteria are constantly seeking to colonise the gut. Bacterial overgrowth is the term given to a disruption of this equilibrium, and micro-organisms (mostly bacterial) that are normal and healthy in the large bowel are then present in the small bowel and other structures. It is a common complication of bowel disease, but may also occur for no reason; particularly in the elderly, where it may be undiagnosed (Zeigler and Cole, 2007). The traditional means of diagnosing this problem is by taking aspirations from the gut (Khoshini *et al.*, 2008). This is an invasive procedure. Several other tests have been developed, such as breath tests, and although these are not yet fully validated, they suggest that this problem may be more common than previously appreciated (Khoshini, *et al.*, 2008).

Helicobacter pylori (*H. pylori*) is a bacterium that we now know can colonise the stomach, an area traditionally thought to be sterile due to its high acidity. This bacterium can only be transmitted from other humans, and if it is present for a long time it may lead to inflammation, dyspepsia and ultimately the development of ulcers within the mucosa and even, possibly, cancer. Early plans to eradicate this organism have been abandoned with the realisation that it is very common, and indeed is endemic in some populations, and so it would be impractical to eradicate it. It would also be unnecessary as most people colonised by it will not become ill with it. People troubled with ulcers from *H. pylori* are treated with antibiotics and the ulcers usually resolve. Antibiotic treatment for dyspepsia is also effective, but the result is less pronounced (Moayyedi *et al.*, 2005). Furthermore there is increasing evidence that *H. pylori* is actually protective against oesophageal adenocarcinoma (McColl, 2007).

> **Activity**
> Consider the patient who you think may have a malabsorption syndrome.
> What might the implications of the syndrome mean for their long-term health?

Structural abnormalities

Short bowel syndrome is the name given to a large group of disorders characterised by an inability to absorb sufficient nutrients, and possibly water. It is usually the result of surgery to remove parts of the gut due to other pathologies, such as IBD. The GI tract is remarkably 'plastic' and if some parts are removed other parts can adapt and nutritional deficiency be avoided: generally short bowel syndrome is said to occur only after about half of the gut has been removed. However, some nutrients are only absorbed at a few specific sites, and if these sites become diseased those specific nutrients may not be absorbed, even though the gut is mostly intact. Thus iron deficiency can occur if the duodenum is removed, and vitamin B_{12} deficiency can occur if the ileum is removed.

Similar problems can occur if the bowel is damaged by radiation to treat cancer, usually of the pelvis or abdomen. Radiation can cause fibrosis and altered vascularisation, and tissues that have a high rate of cell replication, such as the GI tract, are particularly at risk. This is termed radiation enteropathy. When it occurs it is very serious. Radiation has saved the lives of countless cancer patients, but it can be a double-edged sword because of its effects on other local tissues. Larsen *et al.* (2007) estimate that between 5% and 30% of cancer patients experience radiation enteropathy. They followed up 59 such patients: seven (12%) died as a direct result of radiation enteropathy and the deaths of another seven who died were considered to be related to radiation enteropathy. This accounted for nearly one third of the deaths in this group. Radiation techniques are becoming more sophisticated, as are the imaging techniques they rely upon. It is to be expected that radiation will continue to be an important treatment for many patients, but with fewer damaging side-effects.

> **Activity**
> Consider how the patient should be informed about the side effects of radiation therapy. As the nurse in charge of the patient's care, what role do you fulfil in obtaining informed consent? Review Chapter 9 on imaging techniques of the GI tract.

Insufficient digestive agents

Insufficiency of pancreatic enzymes can lead to digestive failure, and can be the result of cystic fibrosis and diseases of the pancreas.

Cystic fibrosis is an inherited condition in which all bodily secretions are altered, rendering them much thicker than usual. It affects about 8,500 people in the UK, making it the most common serious inherited disorder in the country. The most serious effects are seen in the respiratory system. The patient suffers from repeated chest infections, which will often shorten their lives. In the GI tract these thick secretions can cause problems in neonates, when the secretions completely block the lumen of the gut. A dangerous condition called meconium ileus occurs; this requires urgent surgery. From a nutritional point of view, the pancreatic secretions are less effective than normal, and the patient experiences malabsorption and malnutrition. As this is an inherited condition, patients have it from birth and their growth is often impeded and puberty delayed. Chronic malnutrition can cause osteoporosis – thin, delicate bones – to develop. As they get older, the secretion of insulin can be impaired, so that patients develop cystic fibrosis-related diabetes.

The prognosis for people with cystic fibrosis has much improved recently due to greatly enhanced respiratory care; this makes nutritional care all the more important. The person with cystic fibrosis usually requires pancreatic enzymes. These are capsules that are taken before all meals and also before snacks containing fat. They are essential to facilitate the absorption of nutrients. Often patients are additionally advised to take high-energy supplements or specific nutrients that they may require. One group of nutrients that patients often need are the lipid-soluble vitamins. People with cystic fibrosis are at risk of deficiency in these vitamins because a larger than usual proportion of lipid in their diet is not absorbed and so is lost in the stool. Subsequently the lipid soluble vitamins are lost with the stool as well.

Pancreatic enzymes are usually released in an inactive precursor form so that they do not attack the pancreas itself. Pancreatitis occurs when these enzymes attack the pancreas. Pancreatitis can be acute or chronic. Acute pancreatitis is when there is a sudden release of these enzymes into the pancreas causing severe inflammation and tissue damage. Chronic pancreatitis occurs when this attack is less severe but is continual and the pancreas does not get the chance to heal. These situations may be the result of heavy alcohol intake, but can also be secondary to a range of other conditions, including cystic fibrosis and blockage of the bile duct by gallstones. Refer to Chapter 5 for additional information on pancreatitis.

There is a particular problem with alcoholism and nutritional status. Many alcoholics are undernourished, and there are several reasons for this. Alcohol intake appears to increase transport through the digestive tract and also causes a reduction in GI and pancreatic secretions (Morgan, 1982). This is further compounded by liver damage that is common in people who consume significant amounts of alcohol, and that fact that alcohol, which is very rich in energy but deficient in most other nutrients, is often taken instead of nutrient-rich foods. Finally, and ironically, nutritional deficiencies themselves can lead to changes in the intestinal mucosa that further reduce absorption.

Impaired transport

Impaired transport occurs when the lacteals are blocked; perhaps by cancer or tuberculosis (TB).

Assessment

Malabsorption should be suspected if a patient is demonstrating signs of malnutrition when they are eating (or at least attempting to eat) an adequate diet. It should also be suspected in the presence of diarrhoea. The cause of the malabsorption should be identified and, if possible, corrected. Sometimes the cause will be straightforward to deduce; thus if there is a history of IBD it is reasonable to suggest that malabsorption is the result of this disorder. If the cause is not apparent then the patient will require medical tests to identify the underlying pathology. In any event, tests may be required to identify specific nutrients which may be affected. Once a diagnosis has been confirmed every effort will be made to control the underlying pathology. Whilst that is ongoing nursing support will be directed at maximising the nutrients available. This can be achieved through dietary advice or supplementation.

Nutritional status

Table 7.1 summarises some of the key nutritional deficiencies that may be observed in the presence of malabsorption.

Malabsorption is often associated with anaemia. Table 7.1 distinguishes between two types of anaemia, depending on which nutrients are missing. The most common form is iron deficiency anaemia, when the red blood cells are small (microcytic) and pale (hypochromic). This is because many people do not take in enough iron, which is rather difficult to absorb at the best of times, so in the presence of malabsorption iron deficiency anaemia is often the first problem to become apparent. If there is a failure in the synthesis of new cells, as occurs in

Table 7.1 Key nutritional deficiencies in malabsorption.

Symptom	Malabsorbed nutrient
Anaemia (hypochromic, microcytic)	Iron
Anaemia (macrocytic)	Vitamin B_{12}, folate
Bleeding, bruising, petechiae	Vitamins K and C
Carpopedal spasm	Ca, Mg
Oedema	Protein
Glossitis	Vitamins B_2 and B_{12}, folate, niacin, iron
Night blindness	Vitamin A
Pain in limbs, bones, pathologic fractures	K, Mg, Ca, vitamin D
Peripheral neuropathy	Vitamins B_1, B_6, B_{12}

deficiency of folic acid (folate) or vitamin B_{12}, then unusually large red blood cells result – macrocytic anaemia.

Effects of malabsorption within the gut

Many malabsorption syndromes result in the failure to absorb macro-nutrients. Lipid is particularly difficult to absorb, and as it is water-repelling, fat absorption is almost always involved in malabsorption syndromes. This compounds the problems in absorbing vitamins and minerals as unabsorbed fats trap fat-soluble vitamins (A, D, E and K) and possibly some minerals, preventing their absorption and causing further deficiency. The presence of these nutrients in the large bowel can contribute to bacterial overgrowth. One effect of this is an alteration to the bile salts, which are not reabsorbed but instead are deconjugated and dehydroxylated, further limiting the absorption of fats. Unabsorbed bile salts stimulate the colon, causing diarrhoea.

Diarrhoea

The presence of quantities of undigested and unabsorbed nutrients in the large bowel can affect defecation. These materials in the large bowel are osmotically active and cause water to remain in the large bowel so that the contents are increased in quantity and are more fluid, resulting in diarrhoea. The diarrhoea is particularly severe if there is much lipid material in the bowel. This water-repellent material makes the stool loose, offensive and difficult to flush away. Diarrhoea is exhausting for the patient; also the peri-anal skin is at risk of excoriation. The patient may require help to achieve good levels of skin protection.

113

Fluid and electrolyte imbalance

Fluid and electrolyte imbalance is a great risk to any person with diarrhoea, particularly – but not only – if it is accompanied by vomiting. In relation to fluid loss, children and the elderly are most vulnerable to the effects of fluid loss. Usually the large bowel reabsorbs 99% of the fluid that enters it – about 9 or 10 litres daily. The danger of dehydration must not be underestimated, as it can cause the patient's physical condition to deteriorate rapidly and can quite easily lead to death. An assessment must be made of their fluid balance and this must be urgently corrected if required.

Almost as critical as the loss of fluid is the loss of electrolytes. Potassium and sodium in particular can be lost in watery stools. In the first instance this can cause cardiac arrhythmias. In a situation such as this the client will need intravenous sodium chloride, often with the addition of potassium.

Pain

The malabsorption conditions described in this chapter are distressing and debilitating for the sufferer, but they are not usually very painful. The pain they cause is of a colicky nature: slow, grinding and uncomfortable, but not usually agony. Because of that the pain associated with the disorder often does not respond to usual analgesics, but may be helped by obtaining a comfortable position, and also the use of such devices as a heating pad or hot water bottle. Nurses should be alert to erythema ab igne resulting from overuse of such devices.

Activity
What nursing measures would you employ with patients exhibiting erythema ab igne?

Diagnosis

In the first instance the individual's fluid and electrolyte balance needs to be assessed and corrected; possibly as a matter of urgency. Once that is stable, the nurse will want to identify which nutrients are lacking. Energy balance can be estimated by assessing the person's weight, and whether this has altered recently or, in the case of a child, not increased satisfactorily (failure to thrive syndrome).

The patient's protein status can be measured over the short term by assessing nitrogen balance, since most of the nitrogen in the body has come from protein. However, this is of little value in measuring whether they have become deficient in protein over the longer term. For that the nurse may wish to assess the condition of their body tissues, particularly muscle, as this can be affected by protein deficiency. However, lack of use, as often occurs in chronic illness, can also cause muscle atrophy.

Activity
What equipment is required to assess muscle mass?

Lipids are difficult to absorb, so in the presence of malabsorption, lipid deficiency is likely to be present. The key function of lipid is in the provision of energy, as already discussed in this chapter. However, in prolonged malabsorption the patient is likely to be deficient in essential fatty acids, and showing signs of immune dysfunction and an inability to manufacture new cells, and thus unable to lay down new tissue. Iron is difficult to measure directly, but can be estimated from haemoglobin levels and differential blood cell count.

Care planning and nursing interventions
A patient with malabsorption requires a medical and a nursing diagnosis. Once a medical diagnosis is established attempts will be made to correct the malabsorption syndrome. However, this is often not completely achievable, so the nurse will need to address the patient's nutritional status in the long term.

Ideally the patient will achieve satisfactory nutrition by eating well. They should select energy- and nutrient-dense foods, and avoid those foods that may limit absorption, whether by irritating the mucosa of the bowel or by making the nutrients within the bowel more difficult for the enzymes to act on and absorb. Thus many patients will choose a low-fibre diet, as the presence of much indigestible material in the bowel may slow the action of enzymes on the nutrients present. However, such a diet should be adopted with caution, as fibre within the gut can have a positive effect on the regulation and function of the bowel.

The nutrition provided by a well-balanced diet is obviously crucial to patient welfare, but so is the enjoyment of meals, which are often taken with family and friends. The disruptive and demoralising effects of being unable to enjoy a care-free meal, without excessive concern about the effects of that meal on the patient, cannot be underestimated.

Summary

In this chapter malabsorption syndromes have been considered. Malabsorption frequently accompanies systemic illness, and will render the patient weak, debilitated and distressed. Furthermore the person may have fluid and electrolyte imbalances, and these may need correcting as a matter of urgency. If possible the underlying condition will be controlled, but response to any treatment will be less effective if the patient is malnourished, and this may need addressing.

References

Carbonnel, F., Beaugerie, L., Abou, A. R., D'Almagne, H., Rozenbaum, W., Le Quintrec, Y., Gendre, J. P. and Cosnes, J. (1997) Macronutrient intake and malabsorption in HIV infection: a comparison with other malabsorptive states. *Gut*, **41**(6), 805–10.

Carroccio, A., Fontana, M., Spagnuolo, M. I., Zuin, G., Montalto, G., Canani, R. B., Verghi, F., Di Martino, D., Bastoni, K., Buffardi, F. and Guarino, A. (1998) Pancreatic dysfunction and its association with fat malabsorption in HIV infected children. *Gut*, **43**(4), 558–63.

Castaldo. A., Tarallo, L., Palomba, E., Albano, F., Russo, S., Zuin, G., Buffardi, F. and Guarino, A. (1996) Iron deficiency and intestinal malabsorption in HIV disease (1996) *Journal of Pediatric Gastroenterology & Nutrition*, **22**(4), 359–63.

Chun, T. W., Nickle, D. C., Justement, J. S., Meyers, J. H., Roby, G., Hallahan, C. W., Kottilil, S., Moir, S., Mican, J. M., Mullins, J. I., Ward, D. J., Kovacs, J. A., Mannon, P. J. and Fauci, A. S. (2008) Persistence of HIV in gut-associated lymphoid tissue despite long-term antiretroviral therapy. *Journal of Infectious Diseases*, **197**(5), 640–2.

Khoshini, R., Dai, S. C., Lexcano, S. and Pimental, M. (2008) A systematic review of diagnostic tests for small intestinal bacterial overgrowth. *Digestive Diseases and Science*, **53**(6), 1443–54.

Larsen, A., Reitan, J. B., Aase, S. T. and Hauer-Jensen, M. (2007) Long-term prognosis in patients with severe late radiation enteropathy: a prospective cohort study *World Journal Gastroenterology*, **13**(26), 3610–13.

McColl, K. E. (2007) *Helicobacter pylori* and oesophageal cancer – not always protective. *Gut*, **56**(4), 457–9.

Morgan, M. Y. (1982) Alcohol and nutrition. *British Medical Bulletin*, **38**(1), 21–9.

Moayyedi, P., Soo, S., Deeks, J., Delaney, B., Harris, A., Innes, M., Oakes, R., Wilson, S., Roalf, A., Bennet, C. and Forman, D. (2005) Eradication of *Helicobacter pylori* for non-ulcer dyspepsia. *Cochrane Database of Systematic Reviews*, 2005 Jan 25(1):CD002096.

Zeigler, T. R. and Cole, C. R. (2007) Small bowel bacterial overgrowth in adults: a potential contributor to intestinal failure. *Current Gastroenterology Reports*, **9**(6), 463–7.

CHAPTER 8

Intestinal complications of inflammatory bowel disease

Julia Williams

Introduction

This chapter considers the chronic disorder of inflammatory bowel disease (IBD), which typically presents in early adulthood. IBD is not curable, but symptoms are improved by medical or surgical interventions. The person with IBD will experience periods of remission (when the symptoms ease), and relapse (when the symptoms become more severe). The unpredictable nature of the disease results in the person being forced to adapt and live with a chronic illness. This chapter aims to provide a fundamental understanding of IBD, enabling the nurse to assess, plan and deliver immediate care for this patient group. It will also focus on the long-term support required for the person with this chronic, debilitating illness.

By reading this chapter and carrying out the proposed activities you should achieve the following learning outcomes:

- Improve your knowledge of intestinal complications associated with inflammatory bowel disease (IBD)
- Understand the management options available in treating IBD
- Discuss quality of life issues associated with IBD
- Describe the nursing care required when managing patients with IBD

Definitions

The term *inflammatory bowel disease* relates to a chronic inflammation, of unknown origin, affecting the gastrointestinal tract. Individuals diagnosed with IBD experience episodes of relapse and remission, thus leading to an unsettled lifestyle. Two specific conditions are included under the umbrella heading of IBD: Crohn's disease and ulcerative colitis.

Samuel Wilks first used the term ulcerative colitis (UC) in 1859 to describe the inflamed bowel of a young woman at post mortem, and Crohn's disease (CD) was initially recognised as terminal ileitis by Burill Crohn in 1932. The term *indeterminate colitis* was first used by Price (1978) to describe changes identified by histopathologists examining specimens from colectomy: for a small group of patients precise diagnosis was almost impossible to confirm; hence the term *indeterminate*.

IBD is a chronic condition characterised by inflammation and ulceration within the gastrointestinal (GI) tract; ulcerative colitis is commonly found in the large bowel, mostly the rectum. Crohn's disease can affect any part of the GI tract, from the mouth to the anus (NACC, 2010), but most commonly affects the small bowel.

Inflammation of the GI tract caused by other conditions, such as radiation colitis or diversion colitis, is not classified as IBD. A lesser known type of IBD is microscopic colitis; this includes two types of bowel inflammation: collagenous colitis and lymphocytic colitis.

During relapses the characteristics of IBD vary. However, symptoms usually include diarrhoea and abdominal pain. Such symptoms are debilitating to those with this chronic illness. It is estimated that 70–80% of patients respond to standard drugs, whilst the remaining 20–30% respond less well to medical treatment and suffer from chronic, continuous inflammation (Forbes, 2000). When the disease is most severe the patient may require intensive medical treatment or surgical intervention to remove the severely affected area.

It should be noted that IBD is not just a bowel disease. Most patients also experience other problems, which are termed the extra GI manifestations. These include mouth ulcers, joint pain, renal and urinary tract problems, skin problems, ophthalmic complications, hepatobiliary disease, thrombosis and embolism and malignancy.

Epidemiology

IBD is known to affect men and women equally, and onset usually occurs between the ages of 15 and 30 years (Loftus *et al.*, 1998, 2000). However, literature also highlights a late onset of Crohn's disease in those aged 60 years and above (Kyle, 1992). Although its aetiology is still unknown, factors such as immunological disturbances, environmental factors, mycobacterium and genetics have all been identified as possible predisposing factors to the disease (Onnie, 2011). Living with chronic diseases such as Crohn's disease and ulcerative colitis has an impact on patients' lifestyle: even in remission the disease is always present.

Research suggests that IBD occurs more frequently in higher socioeconomic classes compared with lower socioeconomic classes (Sonnenberg, 1990), and more often in urban areas when compared to rural areas (Loftus *et al.*, 2000). As many as 3.6 million people in Europe and the USA suffer from IBD, and it is more common in the industrial world than less developed countries (Karlinger *et al.*, 2000). There is also a higher incidence of IBD in northern Europe and North America compared to Asia and Africa, however the incidence is rising in Asia, North Africa and Latin America (Loftus *et al.*, 2000). The incidence rate in North America ranges from 2.2 to 14.3 per 100,000 inhabitants for ulcerative colitis (Loftus *et al.*, 1998) and 3.1 to 14.6 per 100,000 inhabitants for Crohn's disease (Loftus *et al.*, 2000). Lapidus *et al.* (1997) also highlight that the incidence of IBD is gradually increasing.

The aetiology and pathogenesis of the disease remains unknown: the overall pattern suggests that environmental factors play a significant role, possibly related to economic development and industrialisation (Onnie, 2011). Psychological and social factors are also believed to effect experience of the disease (Maunder, 2005). Cigarette smoking is the most investigated environmental factor associated with IBD, but the effects of smoking on the diseases are different (Sainsbury and Heatley, 2005). It appears that smokers have a lower risk of developing ulcerative colitis. Ex-smokers have an increased risk of developing ulcerative colitis compared to those who never smoked, and in Crohn's disease smoking is a lesser risk factor for developing the disease (Calkins, 1989). Research has also shown that females with IBD who also smoke have a relatively poor quality of life (Probert and Mayberry, 1991). The debate continues as to the effects of passive smoking: Lashner *et al.*, (1993) found that it caused an increased incidence of both Crohn's disease and ulcerative colitis; whilst Lindberg *et al.* (1992) found only an increase in Crohn's disease.

Studies investigating links between diet and disease are particularly difficult to perform (Onnie, 2011), due to poor recall by the respondents and the possibility that respondents had adjusted their diet prior to diagnosis in an attempt to manage the symptoms of IBD. However, the literature does emphasise the importance of diet in the development of IBD; particularly a high intake of carbohydrates leading to Crohn's disease (Riordan *et al.*, 1998), and a high intake of refined sugar, chocolates and cola contributing to the risk of developing Crohn's disease (Porro and Panza, 1985). A high intake of fruit and vegetables and dietary fibre may protect against developing IBD but this remains inconclusive (Reif *et al.*, 1997).

Some research suggests that the removal of the appendix is protective against developing ulcerative colitis (Radford-Smith *et al.*, 2002) whereas others have observed an increase risk of Crohn's disease following appendicectomy (Andersson *et al.*, 2003). What is clear is that IBD is linked to the immune system.

Infectious conditions such as measles and mycobacteria as well as non-steroidal drugs (NSAID) have all been studied in order to explore their links to IBD. Gleeson *et al.* (1994) have reported that either can cause or exacerbate the disease. In the early 1990s there was controversy as to whether the measles immunisation contributed to the development of IBD (Onnie, 2011). A Cochrane Database review found no evidence that measles, mumps and rubella (MMR) vaccination increased the risk of developing IBD (Demicheli *et al.*, 2005), and the early research has now been discredited. Latterly, it has been noted that relatives of people with IBD are more likely to develop the condition themselves (Langmead, 2011), suggesting that a genetic link should also be considered.

Activity
It has been identified that diet may affect the development of IBD, particularly in relation to a high intake of carbohydrates, refined sugar, chocolates and cola. Articulate the advice you would give to patients regarding their diet if you suspected they could be at risk of developing Crohn's disease.

Pathophysiology
Patients with longstanding IBD have an increased risk of developing colorectal cancer, hence the clear guidelines for the surveillance screening of patients who have had their disease for more than ten years (NICE, 2008). Identifying dysplasia early on is pertinent to treatment and management (Carter *et al.*, 2004).

The psychosocial aspect of IBD is of immense importance when managing patients. Sainsbury and Heatley (2005) highlight that there are a number of psychosocial factors to be considered, including gender, socioeconomic status, ethnicity and perceived stress. They recommend all aspects of the individual's life should be considered when planning treatment. Studies show that people with IBD curtail their lifestyles in order to manage their disease (Ghosh and Mitchell, 2007). It has also been noted that people with Crohn's disease suffer from increased levels of depression and anxiety and some people with IBD perceive their illness constrains their personal and professional life (Sainsbury and Heatley, 2005). Clinical features impacting the patient vary depending on the location of the disease, but will include bloody diarrhoea, faecal urgency, abdominal pain, cramps and bloating, and rectal bleeding.

Although ulcerative colitis and Crohn's disease can be similar in presentation, they have very different characteristics. For example, the inflammation in Crohn's disease is transmural (i.e. it involves the full thickness of the intestinal wall) and may involve any part of the GI tract, including the perianal area (Forbes, 2000). Crohn's disease is often complicated by fistulas, abscesses, strictures and perianal disease (Carter *et al.*, 2004). Ulcerative colitis, in contrast, is ulcerative inflammation confined to the colon and/or rectum. Twenty-five per cent of patients experience inflammation only in the rectum, known as proctitis, 55% have inflammation in the rectum, and for 20% of patients the entire large bowel is involved – this is termed pan colitis (Clark, 2011).

Patients with IBD benefit from a multidisciplinary approach in investigating and managing the disease. Diagnosis can be established from history, laboratory and stool tests, and physical, radiological, histological and endoscopic examinations. There are a number of differential diagnoses that should be considered when investigating bloody diarrhoea, such as infectious and malignant causes. Once IBD has been confirmed, disease activity and extent can be monitored with colonoscopy.

Activity

Identify and list members of the interdisciplinary team who should be approached to investigate and manage IBD.

Diagnosis

Endoscopic investigation will include flexible colonoscopy with biopsies. Endoscopy in ulcerative colitis shows continuous inflammation of the colon, whereas in Crohn's disease the inflammation is patchy and its appearance resembles cobblestones. The advent of wireless capsule endoscopy has led to complete visualisation of the gut with minimal risk of complications. Radiology plays an important role in the diagnosis of IBD as it can identify complications associated with the disease. For example, plain X-ray and/or ultrasound will demonstrate the presence of toxic megacolon (a potentially fatal condition of a grossly enlarged colon – over 5 cm – resulting from a loss of muscle tone, with evidence of septicaemia, requiring emergency surgery) as well as confirming the diagnosis. CT scanning and MRI are also useful. Refer to Chapter 9 for additional information on these GI imaging studies.

Blood tests will determine disease activity. For example, raised erythrocyte sedimentation rate (ESR) and/or C-reactive protein (CRP) indicates active disease. An increase in platelets and white cells would indicate infection and chronic disease, and similarly iron studies, showing folate and vitamin B_{12} decrease, might indicate malnutrition. Stool samples are required to eliminate infections such as *Clostridium difficile* (*C.diff*) and are also used as markers at the initial diagnosis or in predicting relapse of disease. Biopsies would be sent for histological examination, further assisting in distinguishing between ulcerative colitis and Crohn's disease.

Activity
Following a review of Chapter 9, describe the preparation of the patient required prior to imaging being undertaken.

Assessment
A thorough assessment is the basis of any clinical intervention; therefore gathering information concerning physical, psychological and social wellbeing offers a baseline record, which in turn complements the investigations, thus facilitating optimum management. Some assessment tools are used to score disease activity in IBD. These include the Simple Clinical Colitis Activity Index (SSCAI) and Harvey–Bradshaw Index (HBI). Effective communication, observation skills and a sound understanding of the disease process are all involved in the assessment of the patient.

Medical management
The major goal of therapy for IBD patients is to decrease or alleviate symptoms and complications, stop the disease progression and maintain a close-to-normal daily life. Modern management of IBD uses a patient-focused approach with the patient at the centre. The modalities of treatment depend upon patient-related factors such as co-morbidities, tolerance, drug interactions, family planning, side-effects and patient preference, as well as disease-related factors such as site and severity of disease, complications and extra-intestinal manifestations. Additionally, funding of treatment must be considered.

Most individuals with ulcerative colitis will be treated with drugs, including 5-ASA therapies such as mesalazine, and steroids, in order to control or reduce the inflammation. Should these therapies fail, steroid-sparing agents, such as azathioprine, should be considered and are often successful in maintaining remission. New biological therapies are currently under development; the most widely known of these being Infliximab (Remicade) and Adalimumab (Humira). Recently in the UK, NICE advocated the use of Infliximab as a rescue therapy but not for chronic active ulcerative colitis, leading to difficulties in obtaining treatment (NICE, 2008).

The drug management for Crohn's disease is similar to that for ulcerative colitis. In addition, various antibiotics can be used. Enteral nutrition plays an important part in the management of Crohn's disease, particularly in children. It can also be a useful alternative to steroid therapy in adults. Successful enteral nutrition requires patient compliance. Most regimens involve taking a large quantity (e.g. 1500–2500 ml over 24 hours) of unpalatable liquid, which many patients find difficult. Nursing support is of the upmost importance. Other treatments include fish oil (omega-3 fatty acids), probiotics, prebiotics, aloe vera, curcumin, and nicotine (for ulcerative colitis only).

Activity

Describe how you would support the patient requiring drug management for Crohn's disease. Identify the nursing actions you would employ that promote patient compliance.

Surgical management

The advent of new medical therapies has greatly improved patients' prospects in acute ulcerative colitis, but it is estimated that 30% of people with ulcerative colitis will still eventually require surgery (Clark, 2011). The aim of surgery is to effect a cure by removing the diseased area of the bowel, minimising complications, retaining GI continuity and achieving the best functional outcome for the patient. Surgery is considered when medical management has failed and the patient is experiencing acute exacerbations of the disease, or in severe symptoms, dysplasia, cancer or toxic megacolon.

Surgery is usually an elective procedure allowing the patient to be part of the decision-making process. Options include panproctocolectomy and permanent ileostomy, total colectomy and ileorectal anastomosis or restorative proctocolectomy (ileo-anal pouch formation). A less frequent procedure is the Kock continent ileostomy (Kock pouch formation). Laparoscopic surgery is now preferred, reducing morbidity and aiding a speedy recovery (Clark, 2011).

Patients with Crohn's disease are even more likely to require surgery – 80% need surgery at some point in their lives, usually due to obstruction or fistula formation – when a tract opens up between the diseased bowel and another part of the bowel or another structure altogether. Such surgery is therefore likely to be elective. The surgery is conservative, meaning that as little bowel as possible is removed. This is particularly important given that Crohn's disease can recur at another site in the bowel. Surgery includes stricturoplasty, drainage and repair of fistula and panproctocolectomy with permanent ileostomy.

Pre-operative care will include a detailed explanation of the surgical procedure using both verbal and written information. Bowel preparation will include restricting fluid intake prior to surgery but will not include a bowel clearance for risk of perforation. If formation of a stoma (ileostomy or colostomy) is to occur it is important that the specialist stoma care nurse see the patient pre-operatively in order to prepare them for the stoma and to locate the stoma on the abdomen for optimum comfort. Anaesthetic assessment and consent are also required.

Post-operative recovery will vary depending upon whether the patient has been entered into an enhanced recovery programme. Such a programme involves avoidance of bowel preparation and pelvic drainage, early oral intake and mobilisation with minimal use of intravenous fluids and analgesics.

The management of the stoma will be taught by the nurse specialist in stoma care and the patient will learn to care for the skin around the stoma and to empty and change the stoma appliance. They will also be alerted to complications associated with stoma surgery and offered support and counselling whilst they adapt and adjust to this new way of living.

Activity
Describe the role of the staff nurse in reinforcing the patient's learning in how to manage their stoma after the patient has been seen by the nurse specialist in stoma care.

Quality of life
Research shows that psychosocial elements and quality of life (QoL) issues play an important role and affect the decisions that are made in treating IBD (Drossman *et al.*, 1989). IBD can lead to impairment of emotional and psychological wellbeing and physical debilitation. The physical and psychological impact of major surgery, and especially formation of a stoma, cannot be underestimated. Whether medically

or surgically managed, IBD has a devastating effect on the patient's QoL. Research has shown that integrating psychosocial care into the medical treatment results in a positive effect on outcomes and improves QoL (Clearfield, 2008). Psychological distress results in increased use of medical services. Furthermore, social factors, such as divorce, death and other stressful events, have been associated with increased disease activity (Williams, 2005).

A good QoL generally means a person can function at home and work, has a good attitude towards life and health, has good relationships, and feels positive about their body. QoL is improved in patients if they are pain-free, can stop steroid treatment, have no complications and have minimal time off work because of their illness.

Activity
QoL is assessed most frequently through the use of Patient Reported Outcome Measures (PROMs) (Whiteing and Cox, 2010). Identify some PROMs that could be used to assess QoL amongst patients with Crohn's disease and/or ulcerative colitis.

Childhood IBD

It is estimated that up to 25% of patients with Crohn's disease and ulcerative colitis are diagnosed prior to the age of 18 (Sawczenko *et al.*, 2001). Although the pathophysiology of IBD does not differ between a child and adult, managing the disease in children does differ and is very important. Children have emotional and developmental needs, which vary with their age and which should be acknowledged when planning treatment. Outcomes deteriorate (risking further complications) if they fail to comply with treatment, perhaps due to lack of understanding or inability to cope. Growth failure has long been recognised as a major complication of IBD in children (Walker-Smith, 1996). Growth is affected by disease activity and treatment, and is therefore an important indicator of wellbeing and a consequent marker for the efficacy of treatment. In relation to the management of growth, children with Crohn's disease are also at particular risk of developing osteopenia (thinning of bones, a precursor to osteoporosis). Prolonged use of corticosteroids has been shown to reduce bone density (Boot *et al.*, 1998). Bone mass should accumulate significantly during puberty; therefore strategies to reduce disease activity then are particularly important.

Treatment using nutritional therapy (i.e. liquid diet), has been shown to reduce inflammation of the gut lining and promote mucosal healing (Fell *et al.*, 2000). Medical management mirrors that of adult management, but monitoring is even more crucial in the effective management of the disease.

Summary

In this chapter the chronic disorder of inflammatory bowel disease (IBD) has been considered. It was identified that Crohn's disease and ulcerative colitis are chronic inflammatory bowel diseases that affect about 1 in 250 people in the UK. Crohn's disease can affect any part of the GI tract, whereas ulcerative colitis only affects the large bowel. The cause of IBD remains unknown, but genetic predisposition is possible and various environmental factors such as smoking and diet may also play a major role. There is evidence that the diseases are increasing.

A patient-centred approach to the management and care of IBD is paramount. Patients need a clear understanding of the disease process in order to assess the risks and benefits of management strategies and ensure compliance. This can often be difficult in a prolonged illness; therefore psychosocial support needs to be ongoing.

References

Andersson, R. E., Olaison, G., Tysk, C. and Ekbom, A. (2003) Appendectomy is followed by increased risk of Crohn's disease. *Gastroenterology*, **124**(1), 40–6.

Boot, A. M., Bouquet, J., Krenning, E. P. and deMuinck Keizer-Schrama, S. M. (1998) Bone mineral density and nutritional status in children with chronic inflammatory bowel disease. *Gut*, **42**(2), 188–94.

Calkins, B. M. (1989) A meta-analysis of the role of smoking in inflammatory bowel disease. *Digestive Disease Science*, **34**(12), 1841–54.

Carter, M. J., Lobo, A. J. and Travis, S. P. (2004) Guidelines for the management of inflammatory bowel disease in adults. *Gut*, **53**(Suppl. 5): V1–V16.

Clark, S. (2011) Surgical management. In: *Inflammatory Bowel Disease Nursing* (eds. K. Whayman, J. Duncan and M. O'Connor). Quay Books, London.

Clearfield, H. R. (2008) How does IBD affect quality of life? *Inflammatory Bowel Disease*, **14**(Suppl. 2), S45–S46.

Demicheli, V., Jefferson, T., Rivetti, A. and Price, D. (2005) Vaccines for measles, mumps and rubella in children. *Cochrane Database Systematic Review*, **2005**(4), CD004407.

Drossman, D. A., Patrick, D. L., Mitchell, C. M., Zagami, E. and Applebaum, M. I. (1989) Health-related quality of life in inflammatory bowel disease. Functional status and patient worries and concerns. *Digestive Diseases Science*, **34**(9), 1379–86.

Fell, J. M., Paintin, M., Arnaud-Battandier, F. Kitching, P., Donnet-Hughes, A., MacDonald, T. T. and Walker-Smith, J. A. (2000) Mucosal healing and a fall in mucosal pro-inflammatory cytokine mRNA induced by a specific oral polymeric diet in paediatric Crohn's disease. *Alimentary Pharmacology Therapy*, **14**(3), 281–9.

Forbes, A. (2000) *A Clinician's Guide to Inflammatory Bowel Disease*. Arnold, London.

Ghosh, S. and Mitchell, R. (2007) Impact of inflammatory bowel disease on quality of life: results of the European Federation of Crohn's and Ulcerative colitis Associations (EFCCA) patient survey. *Journal of Crohn's and Colitis*, **1**(1), 10–20.

Gleeson, M., Ramsey, D., Hutchinson, S., Spencer, D. and Monteith, G. (1994) Colitis associated with non-steroidal anti-inflammatory drugs. *Lancet*, **344**(8928), 1028.

Karlinger, K., Gyorke, T., Mako, E., Mester, A. and Tarjan, Z. (2000) The epidemiology and the pathogenesis of inflammatory bowel disease. *European Journal of Radiology*, **35**(3), 154–67.

Kyle, J. (1992) Crohn's disease in the northeastern and north Isles of Scotland: an epidemiological review. *Gastroenterology*, **103**(2), 392–9.

Langmead, L. (2011) Pathophysiology. In: *Inflammatory Bowel Disease Nursing* (eds. K. Whayman, J. Duncan and M. O'Connor). Quay Books, London.

Lapidus, A., Bernell, O., Hellers, G., Persson, P. G. and Loftberg, R. (1997) Incidence of Crohn's disease in Stockholm County 1955–1989. *Gut*, **41**(4), 480–6.

Lashner, B. A., Shaheen, N. J., Hanauer, S. B. and Kirschner, B. S. (1993) Passive smoking is associated with an increased risk of developing inflammatory bowel disease in children. *American Journal of Gastroenterology*, **88**(3), 356–9.

Lindberg, E., Jarnerot, G. and Huitfeldt, B. (1992) Smoking in Crohn's disease: effect on localization and clinical course. *Gut*, **33**(6), 779–82.

Loftus, E. V., Silverton, M. D., Sandborn, W. J., Tremaine, W. J., Harmsen, W. S. and Zinsmeister, A. R. (1998) Crohn's disease in Olmsted County, Minnesota, 1940–1993: incidence, prevalence and survival. *Gastroenterology*, **114**(6), 1161–8.

Loftus, E. V., Silverstein, M. D., Sandborn, W. J., Tremaine, W. J., Harmsen, W. S. and Zinsmeister, A. R. (2000) Ulcerative colitis in Olmsted County, Minnesota, 1940–1993: incidence, prevalence and survival. *Gut*, **46**(3), 336–43.

Maunder, R. G. (2005) Evidence that stress contributes to inflammatory bowel disease: evaluation, synthesis and future directions. *Inflammatory Bowel Disease*, **11**(6), 600–8.

National Institute for Health and Clinical Excellence (2008) *Ulcerative Colitis (Acute Exacerbations) TA163*. http://www.guidance.nice.org.uk/TA163/140 (accessed January 2011).

Onnie, C. (2011) Epidemiology. In: *Inflammatory Bowel Disease Nursing* (eds. K. Whayman, J. Duncan and M. O'Connor). Quay Books, London.

NACC (2010) http://www.nacc.org.uk/ (accessed May 2011).

Porro, G. B. and Panza, E. (1985) Smoking, sugar and inflammatory bowel disease. *British Medical Journal*, **291**(6500), 971–2.

Price, A. B. (1978) Overlap in the spectrum of non-specific inflammatory bowel disease: colitis indeterminate. *Journal of Clinical Pathology*, **31**(6), 567–77.

Probert, C. S. J. and Mayberry, J. F. (1991) Inflammatory bowel disease: patients' expectations in the 1990s. *Journal of the Royal Society of Medicine*, **84**(3), 131–2.

Radford-Smith, G. L., Edwards, J. E., Purdie, D. M., Pandeya, N., Watson, M., Martin, N. G., Green, A., Newman, B. and Florin, T. H. (2002) Protective role of appendicectomy on onset and severity of ulcerative colitis and Crohn's disease. *Gut*, **51**(6), 808–13.

Reif, S., Klein, I., Lubin, F., Farbstein, M., Hallak, A. and Gilat, T. (1997) Pre-illness dietary factors in inflammatory bowel disease. *Gut*, **40**(6), 754–60.

Riordan, A. M., Ruxton, C. H. and Hunter, J. O. (1998) A review of associations between Crohn's disease and consumption of sugars. *European Journal of Clinical Nutrition*, **52**(4), 229–38.

Sainsbury, A. and Heatley, R. V. (2005) Review article: psychosocial factors in the quality of life of patients with inflammatory bowel disease. *Alimentary Pharmacology and Therapeutics*, **21**(5), 499–508.

Sawczenko, A., Sandhu, B. K. and Logan, R. F., Jenkins, H., Taylor C. J., Mian, S. and Lynn, R. (2001) Prospective survey of childhood inflammatory bowel disease in the British Isles. *Lancet*, **357**(9262), 1093–4.

Sonnenberg, A. (1990) Occupational distribution of inflammatory bowel disease among German employees. *Gut*, **31**(9), 1037–40.

Walker-Smith, J. A. (1996) Management of growth failure in Crohn's disease. *Archives of Diseases of Children*, **75**(4), 351–4.

Whiteing, N. and Cox, C. (2010) PROMs in gastrointestinal nursing. *Journal of Gastrointestinal Nursing*, **8**(5), 16–19.

Williams, J. (2005) Psychological considerations in gastrointestinal nursing. *British Journal of Nursing*, **14**(17), 931–5.

CHAPTER 9

Gastrointestinal imaging studies

Jennifer Edie

Introduction

In this chapter a range of procedures used in imaging the gastrointestinal (GI) tract will be considered. The chapter will give a brief description of each procedure, along with patient preparation and aftercare. It is essential to know that the GI tract can be difficult to image well, as it does not show up clearly on images and the presence of gas and faecal matter can interfere with image quality. The use of contrast agents and good bowel preparation will overcome much of this problem. For these reasons good communication with patients is essential to ensure that they understand the preparation required and what the procedure will involve.

By reading this chapter you should achieve the following learning outcomes:

- Improve your knowledge of procedures used in imaging the GI tract.
- Understand the significance of patient preparation and aftercare.
- Identify the appropriate procedure for assessing and diagnosing problems associated with the GI tract.

Plain abdominal radiography

A radiograph is an image of the internal structures of the body and is produced by exposure to radiation (X-rays) with the image being recorded on a film or in digital form and displayed on a computer screen. Parts of the GI tract may be seen if bowel gas or faecal matter is present, otherwise the plain radiograph may be of limited value in imaging the GI tract. This is because there are fewer contrasting densities, as most of the tissues being imaged are soft tissues. For this reason the use of an abdominal radiograph for diagnosing GI tract problems is not widely undertaken now unless it is to rule out other causes of abdominal problems.

As radiation is used in this examination, female patients who are, or may be, pregnant must inform a member of staff before the procedure is performed. The standard procedure is to take an image of the abdomen with the patient supine; however, an image of the abdomen with the patient sitting or standing may also be taken in those instances where obstruction or perforation may be suspected to see whether fluid levels and free gas are visible.

Activity

Explain the mechanisms you use to communicate to the radiology team that your patient is or may be pregnant.

Fluoroscopy (barium studies)

Fluoroscopy is a procedure which uses radiation to produce a real-time image of parts of the GI tract, where anatomy and function can be assessed. In association with this study a barium contrast agent is used to outline parts of the GI tract which would otherwise not show up well on the images. The main contrast studies are barium swallow, barium meal, small bowel meal/enema and barium enema.

Contrast agents

Barium sulphate suspension is drunk (barium swallow for oesophagus, barium meal for stomach/duodenum) or introduced rectally (barium enema) or via a naso-jejunal (NJ) catheter into the duodenum (small bowel enema). Images are taken with barium coating the mucosa. Air may be introduced to distend organs and to give double-contrast films where the barium shows up as areas of white and air shows up as areas of black on the images.

General preparation for barium studies

To ensure the best possible image quality, the relevant part of the GI tract that is to be imaged must be empty of food/faecal matter. Therefore the patient must not eat or drink anything for several hours beforehand. In addition, the patient having a lower GI tract study may be asked to take a laxative. If the patient takes medicines in the morning, they should not take the morning dose(s), but bring them with them to the X-ray department and talk to a member of staff about whether it is appropriate to take the medicines or wait until after the study has been performed.

If the patient is diabetic and takes oral medication (tablets) or insulin by injection, they need to make sure they have enough to eat on the day before the appointment to prevent low blood sugar. The patient should follow the advice given by the X-ray department. In addition, the patient may be asked to remove some or all of their clothes and to wear a gown during the examination. As radiation is used in this examination, female patients who are, or may be, pregnant must inform a member of staff before the procedure.

Activity
Describe your role in preparing patients for barium studies.

General aftercare for barium studies
The patient will be able to eat and drink normally after the procedure, and should be encouraged to drink plenty of fluids to help the barium pass out of GI tract. The patient's stools will look white and remain discoloured for a day or so after the examination.

The following sections will consider each of the barium investigations in more detail.

Barium swallow
This is a fluoroscopic examination that images the pharynx and oesophagus while the patient is swallowing a barium drink.

- **Contrast agent**: barium sulphate solution to drink, which coats the lining of the oesophagus.
- **Preparation**: Refer to the section in this chapter on general preparation.
- **During the procedure**: the patient will be asked to drink a barium solution and the passage of the barium will be monitored on a television screen whilst images are taken at appropriate times. Initially the patient will be examined standing up and then lying down.
- **After care**: refer to the section in this chapter on general aftercare.

Barium meal
This is a fluoroscopic examination that images the oesophagus, stomach and duodenum.

- **Contrast agents/drugs**:
  - barium sulphate solution
  - effervescent granules (produce CO_2 when swallowed to give double contrast)
  - intravenous Buscopan (to relax smooth muscle and reduce stomach motion)

131

- **Preparation**: refer to the section in this chapter on general preparation.
- **During the procedure**: the patient will be asked to drink the barium solution and will initially be examined standing up and then lying down whilst images are taken. The patient will then be asked to swallow some fizzy granules which produce gas in the stomach and help to show the stomach mucosa more clearly. The patient may also be given intravenous (IV) Buscopan to reduce gut motion. Further images will be taken with the patient lying in different positions to show various aspects of the stomach and duodenum.
- **Aftercare**: in addition to general aftercare mentioned earlier:
  – Some patients may have blurred eyesight for up to 30 min after the Buscopan injection
  – Due to the fizzy gas some patients may feel bloated after the examination

Small bowel meal (SBM)/small bowel enema (SBE)
This is a fluoroscopic examination that images the small bowel (SBM when the barium is taken orally; SBE when the barium is administered via a NJ tube).

- **Contrast agents/drugs**:
  – barium sulphate solution (given orally or ideally via NJ tube)
  – Maxolon (to decrease transit time of barium solution from stomach into small bowel)
- **Preparation**: refer to the section in this chapter on general preparation.
- **During the procedure**:
  – for a small bowel meal the procedure is similar to that for a barium meal but takes longer as additional images are taken while the barium passes through the small bowel.
  – for a small bowel enema a NJ tube is passed via the nose to the duodeno-jejunal flexure and dilute barium is run straight into small bowel and images taken as barium passes through to the large bowel.
- **Aftercare**: refer to the section in this chapter on general aftercare.

Barium enema
This is a fluoroscopic examination that images the large bowel and the barium and air are introduced via a rectal catheter.

- **Contrast agents**:
  – barium sulphate solution administered via rectal catheter
  – air administered via rectal catheter

- **Preparation**: in addition to general preparation mentioned earlier:
  - low residue diet for 48 hours prior to examination
  - laxatives started 24 hours prior to examination (unless contraindicated)
  - no food 6 hours before examination
- **During the procedure**: with the patient lying on their left side the radiologist or radiographer will insert a rectal catheter and the barium liquid is then passed through the tube and into the large bowel. The patient will be asked to move into different positions, both to help the barium pass around the bowel to coat the mucosa and to see other parts of the bowel more clearly. Once sufficient barium is in the bowel, some air is also introduced through the same catheter to expand the bowel further, and improve visualisation of the bowel. Images are taken with the patient lying in different positions.
- **Aftercare**: in addition to general aftercare mentioned earlier, during this examination some patients may feel a mild discomfort from abdominal cramping or pressure due to the barium and gas. When the procedure is finished the rectal catheter is removed and the patient will be able to go to the toilet.

Ultrasound

Ultrasound uses high-frequency sound waves which are directed into the body and the sound is reflected back off internal organs. The echoes are received back and recorded to produce an image of the body. Ultrasound waves do not pass well through air, so ultrasound is not an ideal examination for the GI tract due to the presence of bowel gas, and as such is of limited value for diagnosing the more common bowel problems. It is used more as a first line investigation for generalised abdominal problems in order to rule out non-GI related problems. It has the advantage over plain abdominal radiography of not using radiation. In addition, ultrasound can be useful in cases where pyloric stenosis or acute appendicitis is suspected and where visualisation and measurement of the thickened gut wall can be made.

- **Preparation**: nil by mouth for 4–6 hours to reduce bowel gas.
- **During the procedure**: the patient will lay supine on the examination couch and a water-soluble gel-like substance will be applied to the skin surface so that the ultrasound probe has better contact and moves more smoothly over the skin. The handheld probe which emits the ultrasound is placed on the abdomen and scanned over the skin surface to image the relevant parts of the GI tract. The patient may be asked to move into different positions to help in visualising parts of the abdomen and to help move bowel gas out of the way.
- **Aftercare**: the patient will be able to eat and drink normally after the procedure.

Angiography

Angiography is a procedure where X-rays are used to investigate and image blood vessels and organ perfusion after injecting an iodine-based contrast agent into the vascular system (usually the femoral artery) via a catheter. For the GI tract it is mainly undertaken to image the coeliac axis, superior mesenteric and inferior mesenteric arteries which are the main blood vessels supplying the stomach, small and large bowel. The procedure is done in order to look for GI bleeding, ischaemia or to identify the extent of blood supply to a GI tract tumour.

- **Contrast agents**: a contrast agent is required to allow visualisation of the blood vessels which would otherwise not be seen on the images. For angiographic procedures the agent is an iodine-based fluid. Care is required with these agents as there is a risk in a small percentage of cases of severe adverse reactions to the iodine which may result in anaphylactic shock.
- **Preparation**:
  - The procedure is normally carried out using the femoral artery in the groin for inserting the catheter, so the patient may be asked to shave the skin around this area beforehand. The patient may be given a mild sedative to relieve anxiety if it is felt necessary. The patient will be asked to remove all of their clothes and to wear a gown during the examination.
  - If the patient has any allergies, such as hay fever, or if the patient has had a previous reaction to an intravenous iodine-based contrast agent they must inform a member of staff before the procedure. Informed consent is required for this procedure so checks will be made with the patient about these issues beforehand.
  - As radiation is used in this examination, female patients who are, or may be pregnant, must inform a member of staff before the procedure.
- **During the procedure**:
  - The procedure should be as sterile as possible so the radiologist and other staff may wear a theatre gown and operating gloves. The patient will lie supine on the X-ray table and the skin near the point of insertion, probably the groin, is cleaned with antiseptic, and then the rest of the patient will be covered with sterile theatre drapes.
  - The skin and deeper tissues over the femoral artery will be anaesthetised with local anaesthetic and a small incision made in the skin where the catheter can be inserted into the artery. Fluoroscopic equipment is used to make sure that the catheter is moved into the correct location. The contrast agent is injected through the catheter and X-ray images are taken.

When finished, the catheter will be removed and the incision site closed by placing pressure on the area for approximately 10 to 20 minutes.

– The patient is unlikely to feel the catheter in the artery, but when the contrast agent is injected, they may have a feeling of warmth or a slight burning sensation, which should pass off fairly quickly. The procedure is not painful, but there may be some discomfort from having to remain still for some time.

■ **Aftercare**: the patient will be taken on a trolley to the ward or day-care unit for recovery and observations. Nursing staff on the ward will carry out routine observations, such as pulse and blood pressure, to make sure that there are no problems, and they will also observe the skin entry point to make sure there is no bleeding. The patient will normally stay in bed for a few hours, until they have recovered and may be allowed home on the same day or may remain in hospital overnight. The patient may resume their normal diet after the procedure and will be able to resume all other normal activities 8 to 12 hours after the procedure providing routine observations are normal and there is no bleeding from the puncture site.

Computed tomography scanning (CT)

Computed tomography scanning (CT) provides cross-sectional images of the body using a beam of X-rays which rotate around the patient, and an array of sensors on the other side of the patient that detect the amount of radiation passing through the patient. CT is mainly used to image bowel tumours and for staging. As with other imaging procedures the GI tract is not well visualised on CT scans, so in many cases the patient will be asked to drink a contrast agent to help outline the GI tract.

■ **Contrast agents**: the patient may be asked to drink some contrast agent before the CT scan is performed. The agent should be drunk slowly over a period of one hour prior to the scan (i.e. approximately one cup of contrast agent every 10 minutes) as instructed by the X-ray department staff.

■ **Preparation**:
– to ensure the best possible image quality, the relevant part of the GI tract that is to be imaged must be empty of food. Therefore, the patient must not eat or drink anything for several hours beforehand and for the lower GI tract may be asked to take a laxative. If the patient takes medicines in the morning, they should not take the morning dose(s), but bring them with them to the department and talk to a member of staff there about whether the medication should be taken before or after the procedure.

- As radiation is used in this examination, female patients who are, or may be, pregnant must inform a member of staff before the procedure.
■ **During the procedure**: the CT unit is a doughnut-shaped unit. The patient lies supine on the scan table that is situated in the centre of the unit. During the scan the patient will be required to keep as still as possible and the table (with the patient on it) will move into and out of the scanner unit while the images are taken. The patient will be alone in the room after the procedure begins, but the radiologist and radiographer will watch closely through an observation window. The patient will be able to talk to them through a two-way intercom. CT scanning is not painful, but there may be some discomfort from having to remain still for some time.
■ **Aftercare**: the patient will be able to eat and drink normally after the procedure, and should be encouraged to drink plenty of fluids to help the contrast agent pass out of GI tract.

Magnetic resonance imaging (MRI)

Magnetic resonance imaging (MRI) provides cross-sectional images of the body using powerful magnetic fields and radiofrequency pulses. The MRI machine produces a magnetic field, sends radio waves through the body, and then measures the signal response. The signals produced from the body by this process are used to generate images that are viewed on a computer monitor. MRI does not use X-rays.

■ **Contrast agents**: air in the GI tract acts as a natural contrast agent. Therefore it may not be necessary to use any other contrast agents.
■ **Preparation**: if the patient has claustrophobia they may be offered a mild sedative prior to the scan. Jewellery and other metallic accessories should be removed prior to the MRI scan because they can interfere with the magnetic field of the MRI unit. In most cases, an MRI examination is safe for patients with metal implants; however, the patient must tell a member of staff if they have any medical or electronic devices in their body before the scan in case these are likely to be a problem.
■ **During the procedure**:
   - the MRI unit is a large cylindrical-shaped tube. The patient lies supine on a table that is situated in the centre of the tube. During the scan the patient will be required to keep as still as possible. Like CT scanning MRI is not painful, but there may be some discomfort from having to remain still for some time. The patient may be offered earplugs/ear protectors to

reduce the noise of the MRI scanner, which produces a loud thumping noise during the scan.
  – normally the patient will be alone in the room after the procedure begins. The radiologist and radiographer will watch the patient closely through an observation window. The patient will be able to talk to them through a two-way intercom.
■ **Aftercare**: the patient will be able to leave after the scan has been completed.

Nuclear medicine

Nuclear medicine (radionuclide imaging) uses radiopharmaceuticals to examine how the body and organs function. Depending on the part of the GI tract being imaged the radiopharmaceuticals are either introduced into the vascular system or swallowed and accumulate in the relevant part of the GI tract where it gives off a small amount of radiation as gamma rays. A gamma camera detects this radiation and the images produced give information on the structure and function of the area being investigated. For imaging the GI tract, nuclear medicine is mainly used to investigate gastro-oesophageal reflux and gastrointestinal bleeding. The procedure is different for each of these indications.

■ **Preparation**: preparation of the patient depends on which investigation is being undertaken. For cases of gastro-oesophageal reflux the patient will be required to be nil by mouth 4–6 hours prior to the procedure as they will be drinking during the procedure. For cases of gastrointestinal bleeding the patient will need to have an empty bladder prior to the procedure.
■ **Radiopharmaceutical**:
  – to investigate cases of gastro-oesophageal reflux ^{99m}Tc-DTPA mixed with orange juice is swallowed by the patient prior to the study.
  – to investigate cases of gastrointestinal bleeding ^{99m}Tc- labelled red blood cells are administered by IV injection prior to the study.
■ **During the procedure**:
  – it can take anywhere from several seconds to several days for the radiopharmaceutical to pass through the patient's body and accumulate in the organ or area being studied. As a result, the images may be taken immediately, a few hours later, or even several days after the radiopharmaceutical has been administered.
  – after the radiopharmaceutical has been drunk or injected the patient lies supine on the couch and the camera will be brought close to the body to take the images of the radiation being emitted. The patient may be asked to move into different positions to obtain a clearer image of the area being

studied. The patient may be required to return for more images later in the day or the following day.

■ **Aftercare**: through the natural process of radioactive decay, the small amount of radiopharmaceutical in the body will lose its radioactivity over time. The radiopharmaceutical may also pass out of the body through the urine or stools during the first few hours or days following the procedure. The patient may be instructed to take special precautions after urinating, to flush the toilet twice and to wash their hands thoroughly. The patient should follow any instructions given by the nuclear medicine staff. In addition, the patient should be encouraged to drink plenty of water to help flush the radiopharmaceutical out of the body.

Activity

Write a plan of care for a patient undergoing one of the studies described in this chapter.

Summary

This chapter has considered a range of procedures used in imaging the gastrointestinal (GI) tract and gave a brief description of each procedure, along with patient preparation and aftercare. It was noted that it is essential to know that the GI tract can be difficult to image well as it does not show up clearly on images and that the presence of gas and faecal matter can interfere with image quality. The use of contrast agents and good bowel preparation will overcome much of this problem. For these reasons good communication with the patient is essential to ensure they understand the preparation required and what the procedure will involve.

Bibliography

Chapman, S. and Nakielny, R. (2001) *A Guide to Radiological Procedures*, 4th edn. W. B. Saunders, New York.

Edie, J. (2010) Imaging techniques and clinical investigations. In: *Physical Assessment for Nurses*, 2nd edn (ed. C. Cox), Chapter 16. Wiley-Blackwell, Oxford.

Grainger, R. (2001) *Grainger & Allison's Diagnostic Radiology: a Textbook of Medical Imaging*, 4th edn. Churchill Livingstone, Edinburgh.

Jones, S. (2006) *Imaging for Nurses*. Blackwell, Oxford.

Lisle, D. (2001) *Imaging for Students*, 2nd edn. Arnold Publishers, London.

Patel, P. (2005) *Lecture Notes – Radiology*, 2nd edn. Blackwell Publishing, Oxford.

Royal College of Radiologists *Patient information Leaflets*. http://www.rcr.ac.uk/content.aspx?PageID=323.

Sutherland, R. (2003) *Pocketbook of Radiographic Positioning*, 2nd edn. Churchill Livingstone, Edinburgh.

CHAPTER 10

Other diseases

Warren Chapman

Introduction

This chapter considers other diseases associated with the gastrointestinal tract. Readers of this book will have become aware that the GI tract is a large and complex group of systems. There are many conditions that originate outside of the GI tract, yet their effect is felt within it. The health of the GI tract, in turn, has profound implications on the health and wellbeing of the whole person. This chapter will explore a range of conditions that cannot be neatly categorised as arising within a part of the GI tract, yet still have significant implications for that system. Such diseases include coeliac disease, anorexia nervosa, reactive arthritis, gastrointestinal anthrax and trichinosis.

By reading this chapter and carrying out the proposed activities you should achieve the following learning outcomes:

- Improve your knowledge of other diseases such as coeliac disease, anorexia nervosa, reactive arthritis, gastrointestinal anthrax and trichinosis
- Understand the management options available in treating coeliac disease, anorexia nervosa, reactive arthritis, gastrointestinal anthrax and trichinosis
- Discuss the nursing care required when managing coeliac disease, anorexia nervosa, reactive arthritis, gastrointestinal anthrax and trichinosis

Coeliac disease

Definition

Coeliac (spelt celiac in North America) disease is an autoimmune inflammatory condition affecting the lining (mucosa) of the small intestine. It is induced in susceptible individuals by eating gluten, a protein found in wheat, barley and rye. It has been suggested that the condition developed after the last ice age, when grains were first cultivated in the Middle East (Di Sabatino and Corazza, 2009).

It was recognised in the first and second centuries of the Christian era, while the first clear description and recognition that dietary treatment may be of benefit was provided by Samuel Gee in 1888 (Losowsky, 2008).

Activity
Visit the website of Coeliac UK: http://www.coeliac.org.uk/. It provides excellent information for those with coeliac disease and is a valuable resource for healthcare professionals too.

Epidemiology and pathophysiology

The total number of people suffering with coeliac disease within the UK is estimated to be between 0.5% and 1% of the population (British Society of Gastroenterology (BSG), 2010). The disease can be found throughout Europe, the Middle East, Asia, South America and Asia. The disease has a strong genetic component, stronger than most other complex disorders, and several genes are involved (van Heel *et al.*, 2005). Traditionally, the disease was seen as a condition which presented in childhood, however greater awareness of the disease and better methods of detecting it mean that the there is now an increasing incidence of people diagnosed for the first time as adults.

Gluten gives wheat its baking properties, ensuring the elasticity of dough and allowing it to rise and maintain its shape. In patients with coeliac disease, there is an immune response to a component within the gluten causing inflammation and flattening of villi. This will adversely affect the ability of the small intestine to absorb food and nutrients. Some people with coeliac disease will not suffer any symptoms of the condition until later in life, when an event such as overseas travel, stress, surgery or gastroenteritis will initiate the onset of the disease. It is believed that, once triggered, coeliac disease is a lifelong condition. In patients with untreated coeliac disease, possible complications include osteoporosis, malnutrition (especially vitamin deficiencies), GI lymphoma and increased susceptibility to other autoimmune disease such as diabetes or hypothyroidism (BSG, 2010).

Assessment

Signs and symptoms of coeliac disease can be seen in Table 10.1. Dermatitis herpetifomis is a skin condition associated with coeliac disease: extremely itchy lesions of up to 1 cm in diameter, typically are found on the buttocks, scalp,

Table 10.1 Signs and symptoms of coeliac disease.

- Chronic or intermittent diarrhoea
- Failure to thrive/impaired growth (in children)
- Persistent, unexplained GI symptoms including nausea and vomiting and other irritable bowel syndrome symptoms, e.g. abdominal pain, cramping or distension
- Prolonged fatigue 'tired all the time'
- Sudden or unexpected weight loss
- Anaemia, particularly iron deficiency anaemia
- Dermatitis herpetifomis

elbows or knees, though they can be found on other parts of the body too. Patients may also have a relative who already has a diagnosis of coeliac disease. Many people may themselves already suspect that eating foods containing gluten causes problems. However, the nurse will want to be cautious in assessing individuals, as food allergy can be wrongly blamed for a wide range of problems.

Diagnosis

As coeliac disease can manifest itself in many ways, and can have similar symptoms to irritable bowel syndrome, it can remain undiagnosed unless these symptoms are correctly investigated. In order to aid diagnosis, it is necessary initially to ensure that the patient remains on a diet containing gluten. This is called a gluten challenge. Some individuals may eliminate gluten products from their diet before a positive diagnosis has been proven; however, this can make it difficult to detect the disease. A suitable gluten challenge is 10 g of gluten a day, e.g. four slices of bread per day, for six weeks (BSG, 2010).

The initial test for coeliac disease involves taking blood and checking for antibodies produced by the body against components of the gluten. This is to detect the antibody to the enzymatic component tissue transglutaminase (TTG or t TGA). If the results of the TTG test are uncertain, then a test for endomysial antibodies can be carried out as a second line test – often known as EMA (Hopper *et al.*, 2007). Once serological testing has indicated that coeliac disease may be present, true confirmation of the condition is obtained by taking duodenal biopsies during an upper GI endoscopy. The samples are processed and then examined under a microscope by a histopathologist. Characteristic findings of coeliac disease are blunted or flattened villi along with an increased number of lymphocytes (a class of white blood cells) in the bowel lining (BSG, 2010). Some patients in whom coeliac disease is strongly suspected may have an endoscopy with duodenal biopsy even when serological testing has proved negative.

Care planning and nursing interventions
The treatment for coeliac disease consists of maintaining a gluten-free diet for life. Wheat flour can be found in bread, breakfast cereals, pasta, pizza, biscuits, cakes and many sauces. These can make up a large proportion of dietary intake, so anyone diagnosed with coeliac disease will need a great deal of support in order to maintain a diet that both avoids gluten and ensures adequate nutrition. It is important therefore that such patients are able to see a dietitian experienced in coeliac disease who will give clear advice regarding the correct diet to take. The dietitian may also need to ensure adequate energy intake and supplements of vitamins and calcium.

Patients in the UK with coeliac disease are usually able to have gluten-free foods prescribed. This is important as gluten-free products are often more expensive than conventional foods. The patient's GP will need confirmation of the positive diagnosis of coeliac disease in order to prescribe these foods. As well as wheat, barley and rye, coeliac patients are often advised to avoid oats, as there is a risk that oats can become contaminated with gluten from wheat flour during the milling process. There are oats available which are labelled gluten free and these should be suitable for most people with coeliac disease. Many processed foods and pre-prepared meals may contain traces of gluten. Additionally, eating out may be a problem for those with the disease, as chefs and restaurant staff may not have a good understanding of the requirements of a gluten-free diet.

Patients require follow-up to check that they are complying with the gluten free diet and that it is meeting their nutritional needs. A dual energy X-ray absorptiometry scan (DEXA) will be carried out. This checks the density of bones and so can help detect osteoporosis, a condition which coeliac patients are at particular risk of developing. Regular blood tests will be carried out to check for any vitamin or mineral deficiencies, as well as the function of the liver and thyroid gland.

Some patients' symptoms will not respond to a gluten-free diet. Alternatively, blood levels of TTG or EMA may not improve. Once it has been determined that such people are successfully adhering to the diet and have an adequate understanding of the disease, but their symptoms are not improving, they may require repeat duodenal biopsies. If symptoms persist then other causes will need to be considered, such as lactose intolerance, bacterial overgrowth, pancreatic insufficiency and irritable bowel syndrome. Some patients may need to be referred to specialist centres for management of their condition.

Anorexia nervosa

Definition

The term 'anorexia' originates in the Greek language and means loss of appetite. This may be experienced in many illnesses. The term 'anorexia nervosa' describes an eating disorder: a psychological condition where the individual has an overriding fear of gaining weight and consequently strives for a weight that is unduly low for their age and height.

Epidemiology and pathophysiology

More people die from anorexia nervosa than any other psychological disorder (Hoeck, 2006). Eighty to ninety per cent of patients with anorexia nervosa are female and it has a prevalence of 0.3% in young women. It is also becoming more common amongst young men. The average age of onset in women is 15 years (Morris and Twaddle, 2007).

Many factors are believed to play a role in causing anorexia nervosa. There may be a genetic component and it is believed that the disease may be more common in families where there is a strong focus on perfectionism and competitiveness. It is also believed that social attitudes, which value thin body types, may play a role. Other causes may include childhood developmental problems, negative self-image, educational challenges and family conflicts and other sources of stress. However, the condition does not only occur in dysfunctional families and can be found without any apparent causative factors.

Restricting the amount of calories eaten is only one method that individuals will use to lose weight: they may also utilise excessive exercise to help maintain a lower body weight, induce vomiting after meals and misuse laxatives, enemas, diuretics and slimming aids. Sufferers may also indulge in frequent weighing, self-measuring and looking in the mirror as part of their obsession with their body weight and shape (US National Library of Medicine, 2011; Morris and Twaddle, 2007). Those with anorexia nervosa may go to elaborate lengths to hide the problem from others, including wearing clothes that hide their body shape or eating meals and vomiting afterwards.

Activity

How could you distinguish between a healthy interest in fashion and early anorexia nervosa?

Table 10.2 Signs and symptoms of malnutrition induced by anorexia nervosa.

- Weight loss
- Thin and emaciated appearance
- Amenorrhoea in women (absence of menstrual cycle)
- Poor circulation
- Cold hands and feet and lower body temperature
- Extreme sensitivity to cold.
- Lanugo (a layer of fine hairs covering the body to act as insulation)
- Brittle hair and nails
- Dry skin
- Hair loss from scalp
- Hollow-looking eyes
- Pale skin tone
- Slow heart rate and low blood pressure
- Weakness and tiredness, dizziness, palpitations, chest pain, shortness of breath
- Malnutrition and dehydration
- Constipation and bloating
- Stunted growth (if occurring during adolescence)
- Impaired immunity
- Confusion/poor memory or judgement
- Anaemia
- Swollen joints
- Osteoporosis
- Loss of fertility

The sufferer may well go on to develop signs and symptoms of malnutrition (see Table 10.2).

Diagnosis

Diagnosis will be made through obtaining a history from the patient and their relatives or friends. Furthermore, the presence of any signs and symptoms mentioned in Table 10.2 may assist in assessment. Other causes of weight loss and muscle wasting must be eliminated, such as Addison's disease, coeliac disease and inflammatory bowel disease. Additionally, tests will need to be carried out in order to ascertain the damage that the malnutrition has caused (Table 10.3).

Table 10.3 Additional tests required in the assessment of a patient with anorexia nervosa.

- Dual energy X-ray absorptiometry scan (DEXA) to check for osteoporesis
- Full blood count
- Electrocardiogram (ECG)
- Urea and electrolytes
- Renal function tests
- Liver function tests including albumin
- Thyroid function tests
- Urinalysis

Care planning and nursing interventions

Patients should, wherever possible, be treated on an outpatient basis. Treatment will require interventions to address the eating disorder, as well as management of the physical manifestations of any severe malnutrition. However, sometimes the person is so dangerously ill that admission is required to save life.

Information and support

Patients, families and carers should be given extensive education and information regarding the nature, course and treatment of anorexia nervosa. They should also be informed of self-help and support groups and be encouraged to participate in these.

Activity
Find out what services exist for people with eating disorders in your local area. The NHS Choices website may be a useful starting point. Additionally you may be able to get some information from a dietitian.

Psychological management

Psychological treatments available include cognitive analytic therapy (CAT), cognitive behavioural therapy (CBT) and interpersonal psychotherapy (IPT). The aims of psychological treatment are to encourage weight gain and healthy eating, reduce other symptoms related to the anorexia nervosa and to help physical and psychological recovery. Psychological treatments would be expected to last at least 12 months (National Institute for Clinical Excellence (NICE), 2004).

Pharmacological treatments

Drug treatments alone should not be used in the management of anorexia nervosa. Anti-depressants may be prescribed. The anti-psychotic drug olanzapine may help in reducing anxiety and increasing appetite (Morris and Twaddle, 2007).

Physical management

To correct malnutrition a weight gain of 0.5 kg a week is usually required. In patients who are malnourished it is important that calorie intake is increased gradually, otherwise re-feeding syndrome may occur. Re-feeding syndrome is a metabolic disturbance that can happen in those suffering with malnutrition. As the metabolism in malnourished individuals has adjusted to receiving very little nutrition, the sudden introduction of too great a calorie intake can then cause a disturbance in the body's electrolyte imbalance which can lead to rapid death. Managing weight gain in anorexia nervosa should be carried out in conjunction with a dietitian.

Some patients may require tube feeding via a naso-gastric tube. Very rarely parenteral nutrition (feeding into a vein) is necessary. Occasionally, patients who are deemed to lack capacity may be fed against their will. Such decisions have to be made following the guidance in the Mental Health Act (2007), and will require a court ruling.

Patients with anorexia nervosa may require vitamin and mineral supplements. Additionally, patients who are inducing vomiting should be given advice on dental hygiene as gastric acid can cause damage to the teeth. Advice should include brushing teeth, rinsing with non-acidic mouthwash after vomiting and limiting acidic foods eaten. Pregnant women and those with diabetes will need specific specialised care.

Reactive arthritis

Definition

Reactive arthritis is an inflammation of joints and other tissues following an initial infection, usually in the GI tract (Townes, 2010) or a sexually transmitted infection (STI) in the genitourinary (GU) tract. The condition has been associated with the GI infections including *Shigella*, *Salmonella* and *Campylobacter* and with the STI *Chlamydia trachomotis* (Lozada, 2010). Reactive arthritis has been known as Reiter's syndrome. However, this name should not be used, as Dr Hans

Reiter was not responsible for accurately describing the condition and was also a convicted Nazi war criminal (Keynan and Rimar, 2008), so should not receive positive recognition.

Epidemiology and pathophysiology

Reactive arthritis can affect all age groups but is more common in those aged between 20 and 40 (Lozada, 2010). It is caused most commonly by infections in the GI tract. One to two per cent of those affected by food poisoning may develop the condition (Arthritis Research UK, 2011). Reactive arthritis caused by throat infections or sexually transmitted infections (STIs) is less common. The disease tends to be more severe and long lasting in those with the human leukocyte antigen (HLA)-B27 positive (+) gene; on average 75% of those with reactive arthritis have this gene (Lozada, 2010).

Reactive arthritis typically occurs 2–6 weeks following the initial GI or GU infection. Some patients may not even have noticed symptoms of the initial infection. It is believed that an immune response to the infection leads to the inflammation that can occur in other parts of the body (Lozada, 2010). Inflammation of the joints (arthritis), tendons (tendonitis), tendon insertion site (entesitis), GU tract, eyes (uveitis and allergic conjunctivitis) and skin may occur (Townes, 2010).

The condition will usually resolve spontaneously after 3–12 months but may well recur, particularly in patients with the HLA-B27+ gene. New infections or other stress factors may contribute to recurrence (Lozada, 2010). In addition, the chronic problem of uveitis may develop requiring administration of steroids over a protracted period of time (Cox *et al.*, 2008).

Diagnosis

Diagnosis is made based on the patient history and investigations. Joint inflammation in conjunction with a recent GI or GU infection may indicate the disease. Stool cultures should be taken to check for bacterial infection. In the case of STI, pain on passing urine (dysuria), or a pus-like or watery genital discharge may be experienced. A swab of the urethra should be taken to check for *Chlamydia trachomotis*. Blood tests to check for inflammation (CRP, ESR) may also be taken. Additionally, a blood test can be conducted to check for HLA-B27+ (National Institute of Arthritis and Musculoskeletal and Skin Diseases (NIAMS), 2009).

Care planning and nursing interventions

The initial infection may be treated with appropriate antibiotics. The inflammation may need to be treated with non-steroidal anti-inflammatory drugs (NSAIDS). In

149

chronic cases, drugs which modify the body's immune response may be used, such as sulfasalazine, methotrexate and azathioprine.

Nursing care will consist of managing the symptoms of the condition such as joint pain, dysuria, uveitis and allergic conjunctivitis. Drugs should be administered as prescribed. Fluids should be encouraged for the patient with dysuria. For uveitis, eye drops in the form of steroids (Dexamethasone, 0.1%) and mydrilates (Cyclopentilate 1% or Mydiracyl (Tropicamide) 0.1%) should be given as prescribed.

If the cause of the reactive arthritis is thought to be an STI then appropriate advice regarding safe sex should be given and the patient should be encouraged to inform sexual partners so that they may be tested for an STI. If the cause is believed to be food poisoning then it may be appropriate to offer advice regarding safe storage, cooking and consumption of food.

Gastrointestinal anthrax

Definition
Anthrax is a bacterial infection caused by *Bacillus anthracis* (*B. anthracis*) that usually affects grass-eating animals. It is often fatal for these animals and can be spread to humans who come into contact with infected animals or their products, such as carcasses, meat or skins.

There are three types of anthrax. Cutaneous anthrax is usually spread by wounds in the skin and may be caught by abattoir workers and other people who handle dead animal products. Inhalation anthrax is when the bacterial spores are inhaled into the lungs. Gastrointestinal anthrax can occur if the spores are ingested.

Epidemiology and pathophysiology
It is believed that anthrax may have accounted for the plagues mentioned in the Book of Exodus in the Bible, as well as being responsible for other recorded infectious diseases causing widespread death in humans and animals over centuries (Sirisanthana and Brown, 2002). Anthrax has been found in all continents within tropical and sub-temperate regions. The spores of the bacteria are shed from infected animals into soil. Herbivores may then come into contact with them whilst grazing. Additionally, they may acquire the disease from the bites of specific flies (Cieslak and Eitzen, 1999). Humans may then acquire the disease from the infected animals. Human case rates for anthrax are highest in Africa and Central and Southern Asia. Incidence of person to person transmission is very rare. When humans do contract anthrax it can be fatal, particularly in the inhalational

and GI forms, as it may be diagnosed too late to initiate treatment (World Health Organization, 2008).

Gastrointestinal anthrax can result in severe systematic disease that is fatal in 25–60% of cases. It usually occurs after eating raw or undercooked meat. Immunisation programmes for cattle in the developed world mean that it is rare in these countries (Center for Disease Prevention and Control, 2011). Immunisation is available for humans, but is not routine. However, there has been a recent case of GI anthrax occurring in an unfortunate woman in the USA who came into contact with an animal hide drum which was positive for *B. anthracis* (Mayo *et al.*, 2010).

Anthrax has the potential to be used as a biological weapon, as the spores can be easily distributed. In 2001 spores were distributed through the US mail, resulting in inhalation and cutaneous anthrax causing five deaths (Doganay and Welsby, 2006).

Pathogenesis

In gastrointestinal anthrax, the spores of *B. anthracis* are ingested and cause infection on the surface of the GI tract. There are two types of GI anthrax: oropharyngeal and intestinal. Infection typically starts in the mucosa of the GI tract with ulceration which then spreads to the lymph nodes. The bacteria rapidly multiply in the blood leading to septicaemia. Meningitis can also occur as a result of the infection.

In the oropharyngeal type, a local infection can occur in the throat causing ulceration. A temperature higher than 39 °C may be present. The infection will then spread to lymph nodes in the neck. Symptoms may include severe sore throat, dysphagia (difficulty in swallowing) and swelling of the neck from enlarged lymph nodes.

In the intestinal type, infection can occur in the stomach or bowel wall. Ulceration will usually occur in the ileum and caecum. Those affected may suffer with nausea, anorexia, vomiting and a temperature above 39 °C. These symptoms may progress to very severe abdominal pain, anorexia (loss of appetite), haematemesis (vomiting blood), melaena (black tarry stools containing partially digested blood) or bloody diarrhoea (Beatty *et al.*, 2003).

Diagnosis

Diagnosis may be made by considering the symptoms mentioned above along with a recent history of travel to an area where there is a higher incidence of anthrax. Consumption of raw or undercooked meats will also be relevant. Contact with animal products such as hides should also be considered.

Blood culture samples will be taken to check for the presence of *B. anthracis*. Bloods, to check white blood cell count, erythrocyte sedimentation rate (ESR) and C-reactive protein (CRP), will also be taken to check for evidence of infection and inflammation. In the case of oropharyngeal infection, throat swabs should be taken (NHS, 2011). Cultures of vomit and stool may also be taken to check for infection.

Care planning and nursing interventions

Treatment is with antibiotics, including ciprofloxacin. If deliberate contamination with anthrax is suspected then the Health Protection Agency should be contacted on 020 8200 6868. Vital signs and temperature will need to be monitored closely to monitor for circulatory collapse and response to antibiotics. The level of consciousness should be monitored. Additionally, attention should be paid to signs of meningitis including neck rigidity, rash, photophobia or seizures.

The patient may require analgesia for abdominal pain. Additionally the patient may be vomiting frequently and passing large amounts of liquid stool. Vomit bowls and tissue should be provided and changed frequently as necessary. Appropriate toilet facilities should be provided and the patient assisted with hygiene needs as necessary. Fluid balance should be monitored closely including fluid lost through vomiting and diarrhoea. Intravenous fluids should be given as prescribed and the cannula site monitored and cared for according to the healthcare organisation's guidelines.

The patient with GI anthrax may well have a lot of anxiety about their condition. Furthermore, diarrhoea and vomiting may cause considerable distress and embarrassment. Providing support for the patient and their family will be a key component of nursing care.

Human to human transmission of anthrax is very rare. However, it is advisable to take infection control precautions with linen and bodily fluids as these may be contaminated with anthrax spores.

Activity

Contact your local Infection Control Team and ask them what their guidance is for when patients are suspected to have anthrax.

Trichinosis

Definition

Trichinosis is also known as trichinellosis, trichiniasis or trichinellisasis. It is a disease caused by parasitic roundworm called *trichinella* and is contracted in humans by eating raw or undercooked pork or wild animals. The disease has two phases: an enteral phase and a parenteral phase. There is a high mortality rate of up to 40% (Kaewpitoon *et al.*, 2006).

Epidemiology and pathophysiology

The disease is very rare in the UK (Warriss, 2009), though it can be found in parts of Europe. It is more common in South East Asia; particularly China and Japan.

Humans and other animals can become infected with *trichinella* by eating raw or undercooked pork containing the cysts of the parasite. Once in the stomach the larvae of the *trichinella* are released by digestive enzymes. The larvae then move to the small intestine where they mature into adults and produce more larvae (enteral phase). Larvae pass through the intestinal cells and eventually enter the bloodstream, where they may travel to various tissues in the body including the myocardium (heart muscle), the central nervous system and skeletal muscle (parenteral phase). The larvae entering skeletal muscle form cysts. In affected animals slaughtered for human consumption such as pork, the cysts will not survive if the meat is cooked sufficiently. However, raw or undercooked meat can pass viable cysts on to humans, perpetuating the life cycle of the parasite (Despommier *et al.*, 2005).

The enteral phase corresponds with the larva infesting the small intestine. It lasts about 10 days and is associated with vomiting, diarrhoea and abdominal pain. The following parenteral phase corresponds with the larvae infesting other parts of the body via the bloodstream. During this phase of the infection, the patient may experience pyrexia, myalgia (muscle pain), periorbital haemorrhage (swelling around the eyes) and petechial haemorrhage on the skin, conjunctiva and nail beds.

Diagnosis

Diagnosis is made using a combination of history, examination and blood tests. A history of eating raw/undercooked meat will be relevant along with the particular signs and symptoms mentioned above. Blood tests may show an elevated C-reactive protein and elevated eosinophils. Antibodies can be detected in the blood after two weeks. A definitive diagnosis can be made with a muscle biopsy which may show evidence of the parasite; however it can be difficult to obtain a biopsy which shows such positive evidence (Despommier *et al.*, 2005).

Care planning and nursing interventions

In the initial stage the anthelmintic drug mebendazole may be given. Anthelmintics are drugs which expel parasitic worms from the body. Unfortunately this drug will no longer be effective against trichinosis once the disease has entered the parenteral phase. At this point steroids such as prednisolone may be prescribed (Dupouy-Camet and Murrell, 2007). In the initial enteral phase, nursing care will consist of caring for the patient suffering with nausea and vomiting, as outlined earlier in this chapter for the care of the patient suffering with anthrax.

During the parenteral phase, drugs such as paracetamol may need to be given, as prescribed, to control pyrexia and any muscular pain experienced. Careful observation of skin condition and neurological signs should be maintained and noted. Temperature and vital signs should be monitored. The patient may suffer with dyspnoea and so may need to be sat upright to aid breathing. Oxygen should be given as prescribed and regular mouth care will be necessary. Fluid intake and output should be monitored and intravenous therapy given as prescribed, with appropriate care of intravenous cannula. On recovery, the patient may require education regarding avoiding eating raw or undercooked meats.

Summary

In this chapter a range of conditions that cannot be neatly categorised as arising within a part of the GI tract, yet which still have significant implications for that system, have been considered. The diseases explored included coeliac disease, anorexia nervosa, reactive arthritis, gastrointestinal anthrax and trichinosis. It was noted that the health of the GI tract has profound implications for the health and wellbeing of the whole person and that education regarding the management of many of these conditions is essential for the maintenance of good health.

References

Arthritis Research UK (2011) *Reactive Arthritis* http://www.arthritisresearchuk.org/arthritis_information/arthritis_types__symptoms/reactive_arthritis.aspx (accessed October 2011).

Beatty, M. E., Ashford, D. A., Griffin, P. M., Tauxe, R. V. and Sobel, J. (2003) Gastrointestinal anthrax. Review of the literature. *Archives of Internal Medicine*, **163**(20), 2527–31.

British Society of Gastroenterology (BSG) (2010) *The Management of Adults with Coeliac Disease*. http://www.bsg.org.uk/images/stories/clinical/bsg_coeliac_10.pdf (accessed October 2011).

Center for Disease Control and Prevention (CDC) (2011) *Q & A Gastrointestinal (GI) Anthrax*. http://emergency.cdc.gov/agent/anthrax/gi/ (accessed October 2011).

Cieslak, T. J. and Eitzen, E. M. (1999) Clinical and epidemiologic principles of anthrax. *Emerging infectious Diseases*, **5**(4), 552–5.

Cox, C., Evans, P., Withers, T. and Titmus, K. (2008) The importance of gastrointestinal nurses being HLA-B27 aware. *Journal of Gastrointestinal Nursing*, **6**(9), 32–40.

Despommier, D. D., Gwadz, R. W., Hotez, P. J. and Knirsch, C. A. (2005) *Parasitic Diseases*, 5th edn. Apple Tree Productions, New York.

Di Sabatino, A. and Corazza, G. R. (2009) Coeliac disease. *The Lancet*, **373**(9673), 1480–92.

Doganay, L. and Welsby, P. D. (2006) Anthrax: a disease in waiting. *Postgraduate Medical Journal*, **82**(973), 754–6.

Dupouy-Camet, J. and Murrell, K. D. (2007) FAO/WHO/OIE *Guidelines for the Surveillance, Management, Prevention and Control of Trichinelloisis*. Food and Agriculture Organization of the United Nations (FAO), World Health Organization (WHO) and World Organisation for Animal Health (OIE), Paris.

van Heel, D. A., Hunt, K., Greco, L. and Wijmenga, C. (2005) Genetics in coeliac disease *Best Practice and Research. Clinical Gastroenterology*, **19**(3), 232–9.

Hoeck, H. W. (2006) Incidence, prevalence and mortality of anorexia nervosa and other eating disorders. *Current Opinion in Psychiatry*, **19**(4), 389–94.

Hopper, A. D., Hadjivassilou, M., Butt, S. and Sanders, D. S. (2007) Adult Coeliac Disease. *British Medical Journal*, **335**(7619), 558–62.

Kaewpitoon, N., Kaewpitoon, S. J., Philasri, C., Leksomboon, R., Maneenin, C., Sirilaph, S. and Pengsaa, P. (2006) Trichinosis: epidemiology in Thailand. *World Journal of Gastroenterology*, **12**(40), 6440–5.

Keynan, Y. and Rimar, D. (2008) Reactive arthritis – the appropriate name. *Israel Medical Association Journal*, **10**(4), 256–8.

Losowsky, M. S. (2008) A history of coeliac disease. *Digestive Diseases*, **26**(2), 112–20.

Lozada C. J. (2010) *Reactive Arthritis*. http://emedicine.medscape.com/article/331347-overview (accessed October 2011).

Mental Health Act (2007) http://www.legislation.gov.uk/ukpga/2007/12/contents (accessed September 2011).

Mayo, L. *et al.* (2010) Gastrointestinal Anthrax after an Animal-Hide Drumming Event – New Hampshire and Massachusetts, 2009. Center for Disease Control and Prevention. http://www.cdc.gov/mmwr/preview/mmwrhtml/mm5928a3.htm (accessed October 2011).

Morris, J. and Twaddle, S. (2007) Anorexia nervosa. *British Medical Journal*, **334**(7599), 894–8.

NHS (2011) *Anthrax – Suspected. Map of Medicine*. NHS Institute for Innovation and Improvement. http://eng.mapofmedicine.com/evidence/map/anthrax1.html (accessed October 2011).

National Institute for Clinical Excellence (NICE) (2004) *Clinical Guideline 9. Eating Disorders. Core Interventions in the Treatment and Management of Anorexia Ner-*

vosa, Bulimia Nervosa and Related Eating Disorders. http://www.nice.org.uk/cg-009niceguideline (accessed October 2011)

National Institute of Arthritis and Musculoskeletal and Skin Diseases (NIAMS) (2009) *Reactive Arthritis*. http://www.niams.nih.gov/Health_Info/Reactive_Arthritis/default.asp (accessed October 2011).

Sirisanthana, T. and Brown, A. E. (2002) Anthrax of the gastrointestinal tract. *Emerging Gastrointestinal Diseases*, **8**(7), 649–51.

Townes, J. M. (2010) Reactive arthritis after enteric infections in the United States: the problem of definition. *Clinical Infectious Disease*, **50**(2), 247–54.

US National Library of Medicine (2011) *Anorexia Nervosa*. http://www.nlm.nih.gov/medlineplus/ency/article/000362.htm (accessed October 2011)

Warriss, P. D. (2009) *Meat Science: An Introductory Text*, 2nd edn. CABI, Oxford.

World Health Organization (2008) *Anthrax in Humans and Animals*, 4th edn. http://www.who.int/csr/resources/publications/anthrax_webs.pdf (accessed October 2011).

Index